HISTORY OF PSYCHOLOGY AND PSYCHIATRY

by A. A. Roback

GREENWOOD PRESS, PUBLISHERS
NEW YORK

First Greenwood Reprinting 1969

Library of Congress Catalogue Card Number 71-88929

SBN 8371-2104-3

PRINTED IN UNITED STATES OF AMERICA

HISTORY OF PSYCHOLOGY AND PSYCHIATRY

PREFACE

While not intended as a complete history, it is hoped that the volume will serve to point out and describe the milestones in the progress of the mental sciences, in sequence. Wherever the topic lent itself to direct quotation from an author, significant passages were reproduced, so that this work is in part an anthology.

In the majority of cases, primary sources were consulted, resulting in protracted labors over years. It was my purpose especially to bring out some little-known facts in the course of the development of both psychology and psychiatry. Many tributaries fall into the large stream, some of which are not taken account of by the historians, who are intent upon dwelling on the more accessible currents.

American psychologists who will miss sketches of living psychologists (an exception was made for two or three (who are over 80,) in the United States, and half a dozen abroad) must remember that once the sluice gates are opened for our contemporaries, we should have to include at least hundreds out of the 25,000 productive psychologists and psychiatrists, a large number of them specialists in this or that field. How could one do justice to each without expanding the work into an encyclopedia? Hence, it was thought best to list some twoscore of eminent living representatives and admit that a few scores of others may have been chosen in addition.

Questions will naturally arise in the minds of the

trained reader as to why this or that topic had received so much space. It is obvious that such queries, even if anticipated, cannot be discussed and answered to the satisfaction of cavillers. Suffice it to say that the plan was thought out carefully and serious deliberation was given to the problems of inclusion and exclusion. As a rule, priority was given to originators, pioneers, rather than to elaborators. Historical aspects were treated generally under the head of the individuals who were directly connected with the events, on the basis that the *Zeitgeist* is no volcanic eruption or something which evolves "out of thin air"; and in the conviction that what has been "in the air" had first been brewing under the hair. That an idea is relayed and improved upon goes without saying, but eons of time, without a germinating mind, will not discover thermodynamic laws, nor formulate the quantum theory or principle of relativity.

Cambridge, Mass. A. A. Roback

CONTENTS

Part II. Abnormal and Medical Psychology

Part I

GENERAL PSYCHOLOGY

A
THE ROOTS AND TRUNK

ARISTOTLE (384-322 B.C.)—The Great Realist

While the maxim "Know thyself" had been attributed to even the early Thales long before it was attached to Socrates' name, and speculation about the soul, its composition, and its movements, had been rife among the pre-Socratics, broadening and deepening with Plato, in the course of his dialogues; it was nevertheless the Stagirite, probably the greatest synthetic mind in antiquity, if not of all time, who wrote the first treatise on psychology, which is usually referred to by the Latin title, *De Anima.*

This work not only surveys the thought of his predecessors but builds up an analytic psychology, which might be considered the first textbook on the subject. His starting-point is always the definition, and although he proceeds, for the most part in armchair fashion to theorize and argue his point, it is most astonishing to find him clarifying the data on the various sensations and sense qualities in a thoroughly modern procedure. It is evident from his various writings on psychology that, aside from observation, Aristotle had experimented on the senses, else he could not have alluded to positive after-images or to the media of the senses (air, water).

It is true that Aristotle is still preoccupied with the so-called elements (air, fire, water, earth) and many of his explanations are in terms of dry and moist —a conception which was taken over by his followers as late as the Renaissance. Still more curious is his citing as fact the belief that "when women look into a very clear mirror after menstruation, the mirror's surface will be seen covered by a reddish mist." Of greater interest to us is his elaborate explanation of this questionable phenomenon.

Aristotle's contribution to psychology is immense—not restricted by any means to the double-object illusion which carries his name.

His chief "boner" is his placing the soul as the source of thought in the heart, as the *heat-generating* organ. This was in line with the Biblical phrase, "the thoughts of his heart." Plato in that respect followed the Sicilian School, which was regarded as "lowbrow" by the great Aristotle, and thus, for once, the semi-mystical Plato, in espousing the new-fangled theory that the highest soul was located in the brain, scored a point on the scientist and realist.

PLATO (429-348 B.C.) The Idealist

It is difficult to say which was the greater genius —Aristotle or Plato. They certainly had different types of mind. Both are great as philosophers. Aristotle's emphasis was upon science, while Plato's imagination savored of the poetic. Hence Aristotle was the more objective of the two. It was fortunate, however, that Plato came first and that Aristotle was brought under his tutelage at the Academy about 400 B.C. Had it been the other way around, we might have missed in the Stagirite the breadth of mind that is evident in almost everything he wrote. While he did not choose Plato's dialectic method, which was a heritage of the Sophists, he could not but have felt the impact of his master's powerful logic and the extent of the goals at which he was aiming.

Aristotle and Plato started from different points of departure. The former observed a phenomenon and analyzed it, and set it beside other phenomena, thus building up a system, somewhat in the way Wundt and Titchener, thousands of years later, attempted to do in their structural psychology. Plato, on the other hand, was a primitive functionalist. He saw things in the whole, always asked the question, "To what purpose?"

Thus, we may say that Aristotle was the theoretician for whom even the *summum bonum* in ethics is *contemplation,* while Plato is always concerned with the practical. With all his imaginativeness and seemingly unrealistic conception of the substantiality of Ideas or Forms, reversing the common-sense view that qualities only attach to tangible things in the abstract, he nevertheless moves constantly in a practical world. His characters are alive, his analogies instinct with action. Even his metaphysics is teleological; and perhaps every one of his dialogues can be shown to serve the purpose of obtaining guidance in ordering the state of our own life.

The modern experimenter proceeds on the basis of some hypothesis. Plato, although he does not tell us whither he is bound, knows beforehand what the conclusion is going to be, and leads the argument, often through the repeated concessions of a stooge, in the direction of his objective.

In this manner, he highlights a number of midway stations, but they are only secondary stages. What he envisions finally is the state. Everything else must harmonize so as to lead up to its perfect functioning. Hence the individual is just a unit in the larger whole, and his functions are really minor expressions of its over-all functions.

Plato's psychology is, hence, subordinate to his philosophy of the state and to social ethics. It must necessarily be fragmentary. Aristotle, on the other hand, gave us practically a textbook, dealing with all the major mental processes; sensations, perceptions, emotions, etc., following the course of his observations, which occasionally invited experimentation.

Plato was no experimenter; and even his everyday observations were overcast with thought, with intuitions that fitted into the scheme of his philosophical panorama. Both Aristotle and Plato had recourse, naturally, to introspection, which was tinged with interpretation and explanation, similar to a child who, instead of drawing the top of a glass as an ellipse, "sees" it as a circle.

Plato's chief contribution—perhaps his only contribution—to psychology is his conception of the soul. Whether its tripartite division was original with him or was derived from Egyptian and Eastern lore, which had always impressed him, the concept seems to have taken, and held its ground even to our own day. His intuition, which he calls in *The Republic* "the eye of thought," sometimes stood him in good stead, as when he placed thought in the head, instead of the heart, as did Aristotle and the Bible ("He said in his heart"). The *logistikón nous,* which he equated with the brain, is, by virtue of its rational function, the higher phase. Today, it would correspond to the cortex, which mediates cognition and reasoning.

For him the soul, which represents the active emotions—spiritedness, rather than spirituality—resides in the chest. The Greek word *thumós,* which might be translated "courage" and would include valiancy, grit, resolution, will power, and stamina, can also refer to striving, aspiration, and is thus in a sense analogous to our term "conation." It is curious that the German *Mut,* although a palindrome of *thum* (*ós*), corresponds to it exactly.

The third phase of the soul, associated with the lower part of the abdomen, is supposedly non-rational (*alogistikón*) and represents the appetitive instincts in man (*'epithumetikon*). Here are located all the desires, passions, lusts. But love in the higher, more poetic sense (*eros*) is assigned to the middle section —the chest, where the active emotions originate.

It may be possible to subdivide each of these phases into a theoretical and practical category. Furthermore, they may be paired with the four types of cognition: (a) pure reason (*noesis*); (b) understanding (*dianoía*); (c) belief based on opinion (*dóxa*); and (d) conjecture (*ekasía*).

To Plato, the body was sort of a dungeon, and the soul its governor. Without elaborating on his highly ingenious doctrine of the soul, suffice it to say that some elements of it still live in modern psychology. We can spot them, for example, in Freud's topographical division of the psyche, where the id would correspond to Plato's appetitive soul; the ego to the *thumós*, the striving, realistic, ambitious and also fighting and parrying part of our nature; and finally the superego, the *ego*-ideal, which gives rise to conscience, guilt feelings, and spirituality, to Plato's pure reasoning soul. True, the superego in Freud's psychology is hardly a reasoner, being beset by irrational cast-offs from the id, and from a hygienic or clinical angle inferior to the ego, but to many of the para-Freudians and the ethical, in general, the superego should be the last tribunal, even if it hurts.

Jung is even more beholden to Plato. Indeed, it may be said of him that he is a twentieth-century Platonist. The doctrine of the collective unconscious is more than hinted at in *The Republic,* while the theory of archetypes, which figures so prominently in Jung's analytic psychology (the name is a misnomer, for Jung never analyzes, but rather intuits, in the manner of the Greek master), is a basic Platonic tenet, accounting for the memory of the Ideas which but for the soul we could not have. The archetypes or, as Plato called them, *paradeigmata,* are supposedly external, and through them the soul recognizes things, which are copies of the Ideas.

We see, accordingly, that Plato has been the source of greater stimulation than one might expect, and that his seemingly topsy-turvy system of making real entities out of abstract notions and turning palpable objects like stones, tables, or trees into mere copies has not been dumped entirely into the limbo of historical fantasies. The two Greek colossi, whose divergent world views dominated the world's thought for well nigh two thousand years, each appealed to a different philosophic temperament, and served as complements to one another. Reincarnations of their doctrines will continue to appear in modern guise, adjusted to the *Zeitgeist.*

TERTULLIAN (*c.* 150-221)— First Christian Psychologist

The first Christian psychologist was the fiery Church Father, Tertullian, whose range of knowledge, particularly in the field of history and philosophy, was immense. The son of a Roman military officer stationed in Carthage, he received an excellent education and after living the self-indulgent life of the Roman middle class for years, he became a Christian and probably the chief of Christian apologists. A rhetorician of unusual powers, he minced no words in dealing with his opponents, his chief weapon being mordant wit.

His argumentation is marked by great subtlety of expression and an intransigence which gives his adversary no quarter, but his tactics are not altogether fair; for he will on occasion introduce anecdotes and wild gossip and then proceed to abuse his target, whether it is Socrates, Plato, or Pythagoras. He even applies epithets equivalent to our "dumb cluck" or "muddlehead." His approach, although his diction is immeasurably superior, reminds one of our better-known hard-hitting columnists. In his essay "On the Soul," for instance, in controverting the doctrine of transmigration, he has this to say about a certain Ennius. "Ennius once dreamed that Homer had lived in the body of a peacock. Now I wouldn't believe a poet even when he was awake, though I do admit that a peacock is a beautiful bird and none has more beautiful tail feathers. But since a poet's joy is in singing his songs, what good is a handsome tail when he has a raucous voice?" Speaking of Simon of Samaria, whose apocryphal or merely mythical adventures he passes in review, he has this to say in apostrophic fashion:

> However, it was not for you alone, Simon, that they invented this theory of transmigration of souls. Carpocrates naturally made good use of it, too, and he is just like you, a magician and a fornicator, except that he had no Helen. He believed that souls continued to take new bodies in order to accomplish the complete overthrow of all human and divine truth. He held that no man's life was utterly complete until he had befouled himself with every iniquity that is considered vile. You see, he held that nothing was really bad but thinking makes it so. Hence, transmigration was demanded if any man in the first stage of life has not indulged in all that is forbidden. For, obviously, sin is the natural product of life! So, the soul had to be called back to life if it were found below the quota of sin, 'until it has paid the last farthing' and is cast into the prison of the body.[1]

We can well imagine that a man with such a temperament would not curry favor with the authorities, even in his own sphere. As he was accumulating victims of his spleen, he began to find himself quite lonely, and turned to the Montanists, who practiced a rigid asceticism and were given to ecstatic spells, which appealed to a semi-mystic and emotional mind like Tertullian's. To many, Tertullian is known because of his oft-quoted dictum "*Credo quia absurdum est*" ("I believe it because it is absurd"), which is usually misinterpreted, but his writings are marked by a logical temper, although frequently marred by irrelevant old wives' tales and Scriptural crutches.

Because he embraced the heretical doctrine of the Montanists, his place among the Church Fathers was for centuries insecure, though his brilliancy could never be denied—his intellect even transcending in that respect, perhaps, although not in depth, that of his greater townsman (for Tagaste was practically a suburb of Carthage) St. Augustine.

What were Tertullian's views on the soul? In the first place, he polemicizes against Plato, who taught that the soul was incorporeal. Tertullian was certain that it was corporeal, although not of the same stuff as the body. Taking the Bible as his authority, Tertullian concludes that the soul is the breath of God, as the origin of the word "spirit" suggests, yet he cautions us against regarding it as spiritual, in the sense of incorporeal. Like Klages, of our own time, he insists on the dichotomy between mind and soul, the latter being superior. The soul, he holds, is present in the tiniest embryo, and is coeval with the body formation. Dreams are explained by the activity of the soul, which "wanders over land and sea, engages in trade, is excited, labors, plays, sorrows and rejoices, pursues the lawful and the unlawful and clearly shows that it can accomplish much without the body" for "in sleep, the soul acts as if it were present elsewhere."

He differs from Plato also in regard to the seat of the *psyche;* like Aristotle, he believes it is lodged in the heart, again taking his cue from verses in the Bible.

ST. AUGUSTINE (354-430)

Between Galen [1] and Thomas Aquinas there was only one man in the early Middle Ages worthy of inclusion in our survey, and he was a titan, considered the greatest of the Church Fathers, and as a personality, fascinating enough to serve as the hero of a Hollywood film.

Born of a pagan father and a Christian mother in Numidia, Africa, he was brought up by the best tutors; but being a rich boy, he behaved much as teen-agers of prosperous homes behave today. He chose his companions for their conviviality; and fun-loving as he was, he formed a liaison with a young woman who bore him a son. Like the average adolescent, he even stole some fruit just for the deviltry of it.

With all his capers, he nevertheless differed from his pals in that he kept amassing knowledge, and sharpened his intellect until in his late twenties he was in line for a professorship; and as he was entering his thirtieth year, he became the incumbent of the chair in rhetoric (which was then an important discipline, comprising more than the use of language in forensics) at the University of Milan, a very important institution at the time.

It was here that he met St. Ambrose, Bishop of Milan, and under his influence was converted to Christianity. At the age of thirty-two, together with his illegitimate son, who was close to his heart, he was baptized, and such a hold did his mother's religion take on him that he decided to give up his academic position, and returning to Tagaste, his native place, he formed a small semi-monastic center. On one occasion he visited Hippo, which was close to Carthage, for a conference. There he met the Bishop of Hippo, and later was prevailed upon by the Christian community to become a presbyter of the Church. Soon he became coadjutor to the Bishop, and upon the death of his superior, young as he was, he filled the vacant bishopric. His death occurred in Hippo just as the Vandals were besieging the city, prior to sacking and ruining it.

Of Augustine's voluminous works, which would fill a couple of shelves, his *De Civitate Dei* ranks as the most solid. In the *City of God,* we find an apologia of Christianity and a theodicy, according to which perfection needs a certain amount of evil to complement it. His views were a mixture of Platonism and Paulinism, and he laid down the dogma of absolute predestination but irresistible grace. He was an anti-intellectualist, resting his theory on a supernaturalism which became the vogue in medieval philosophy until the time of St. Thomas Aquinas, who favored Aristotle.

A work which will live through the ages is his *Confessions,* in which he recounts his moral and mental development, dwelling on his youthful escapades, temptations, frustrations, and deliverance thanks to Providence. It is probably the first psychological autobiography on record, and divested of the apostrophes to God, to whom these self-acknowledgments are made as an offering, the book contains a mass of data valuable from many angles, but especially from the psychological. It is a literary masterpiece, in spite of the numerous protestations of love for God, which smack of a mawkish sentimentality.

In St. Augustine, there is a curious mixture of

naïveté and sophistication, of impetuosity and deliberateness, of exhibitionism and self-criticism. He asks why he need tell God of all his doings in the past since God is omniscient, and as for his motives in revealing them to others, he has this to say:

> But, what business have I with men that they should hear my confessions, as if they could become the healers 'of all my diseases?' A race interested in finding out about the other man's life, slothful in amending their own! Why do they seek to hear from me what I am, when they do not wish to hear from Thee what they are? And how do they know whether I am telling the truth when they hear about me from myself, since no one 'among men knows what goes on in a man, save the spirit of the man which is in him?' But, if they hear about themselves from Thee, they cannot say: 'the Lord is lying.' For, what is it to hear about oneself from Thee, but to know oneself? Who, then, can know himself and say: 'It is false,' unless he himself lies? But, because 'charity believes all things,' certainly among those whom it makes one, in intimate union with each other, I, also, O Lord, do even confess to Thee in such a way that men may hear, though I cannot prove to them that the things I confess are true. But, they whose ears charity doth open unto me, they believe me.

Throughout his confession, he manages to discuss many psychological topics—memory, imagination, will, sense impressions—but his intricate and profound treatment of time, in which the empiristic and nativistic issues are threshed out some 1,550 years ago, attests as much as anything to his mental acumen and grasp of problems, even though he sees them ever through the theological prism. He is always seeking

God's aid to enlighten him on all matters which puzzle him, and he is constantly drawing on the Scriptures, mainly Paul's Epistles, to bolster his viewpoint. His arguments are often dialectical, and he occasionally introduces paradox, perhaps because of the duality of his nature, a blend of mysticism and rationalism. A sample of his argumentation is in order at this point.

> So, I said, a little while ago, that, as periods of time are passing by, we measure them, being thus able to say that this period of time is double that single one, or this is just as long as that, and whatever else we can express by measuring concerning the relationship of the parts of time.
>
> For this reason, as I was saying, we do measure periods of time as they are passing by. If anyone say to me: 'How do you know this?' I may reply: 'I know, because we do measure them, and we cannot measure things which do not exist, yet past and future things do not exist.' But, how do we measure present time, when it has no length? Therefore, it is measured as it is passing by. When it has passed away, it is not measured; for, what might be measured will not then exist.
>
> But, whence, by what way, and whither does it pass, when it is measured? Whence, but from the future? By what means, but through the present? Whither, if not into the past? From that, then, which does not yet exist, through that which is without length, into that which is already out of existence.
>
> But, what do we measure, if not time in some length? For, we cannot talk about single, double, triple, and equal periods—and whatever else we say about time in this way—except in terms of lengths of time. In what length, then, do we measure time as it is passing away? Is it in

the future, from which it is passing?[2] But, we do not measure what does not yet exist. Is it in the present, by which it is passing? But, we do not measure a thing of no length. Is it in the past, to which it is passing? But, we do not measure what is already out of existence.[3]

THOMAS AQUINAS (1225-1274)

Known as "Doctor Angelicus," chief pillar of Catholic thought, Aquinas served as a beacon light for Scholastics through seven centuries. Dying at the age of forty-nine, he left behind a long shelf of books, chief of which is his voluminous *Summa Theologica,* comprising not only an ontological system, but a miniature interpretative psychology and sociology. A follower of Aristotle, he codified and applied psychological observations to practical life in keeping with Church dogma and on Aristotelian principles. Faculty psychology was first systematized by Thomas Aquinas. There are three grades of the soul, five genera of faculties, and each of the faculties, except the locomotive, is subdivided into species. Status of any operation or deed is determined according to act and purpose. Thus copulation can be of a spiritual nature if the object is reproduction; but sensual if it stems from the lower order of the vegetative faculty.

JUAN LUIS VIVES (1492-1540)—An Original Psychologist

Born in one of the most eventful years in history, at a time when Spain was at the zenith of its glory, Vives represents humanism at its best, together with Reuchlin, Melanchthon, Erasmus, and Thomas More. It was through the latter that he became a sort of court counselor and private secretary of Catherine of Aragon, whom Henry VIII later divorced, whereupon Vives, because he sided with the Queen, was forced to leave England after a brief incarceration.

The foe of empty formalism and dogmatic scholasticism, he became a relentless critic of the prevailing system of education; and his place in the history of pedagogy cannot be disputed. His theological and political writings have exercised considerable influence, but if he is rated as one of Spain's foremost philosophers, it is largely because of the fame he achieved through his *De Anima et Vita*, which came out two years before his death. Within the next two centuries, fully a dozen editions appeared in various countries, some in his collected works. Of contemporaneous psychological works, only Amerbach's treatise of 1542, and Melanchthon's *Commentarius de Anima* can be mentioned in the same breath, although the former was decidedly a derivative of Aristotle's great work.

In his classification, his taxonomy, and biological orientation, Vives leans much on both Aristotle and Galen. The selection of topics is naturally conditioned

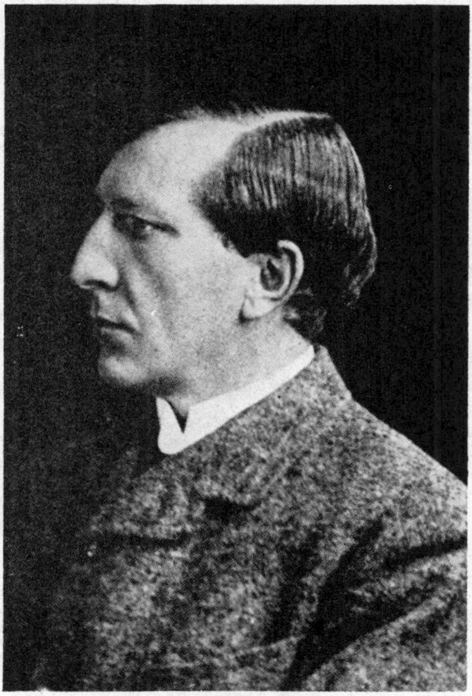

William McDougall

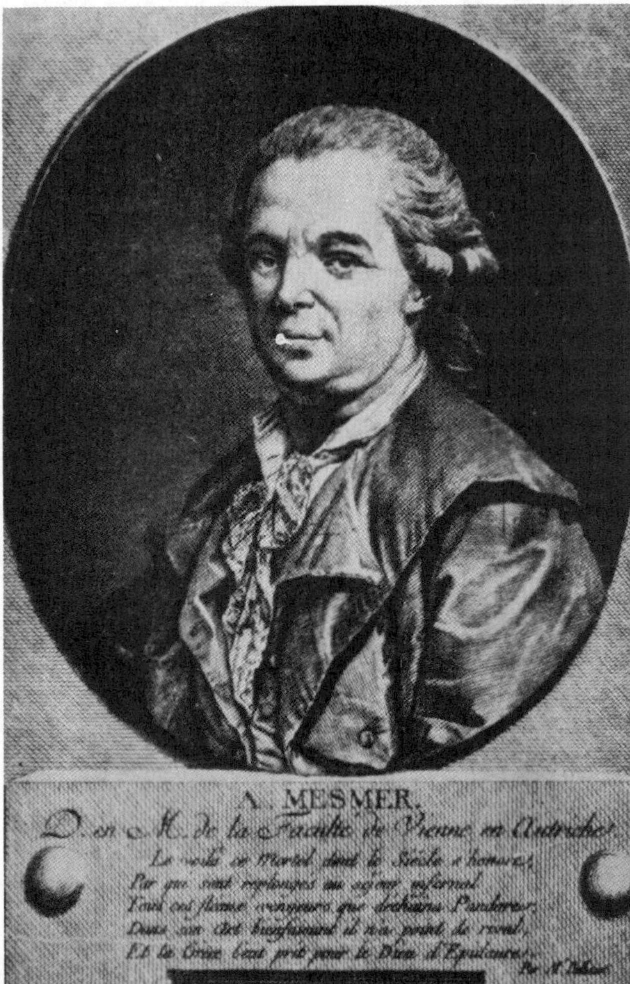
A. MESMER.
D. en M. de la Faculté de Vienne en Autriche.

Anton Mesmer

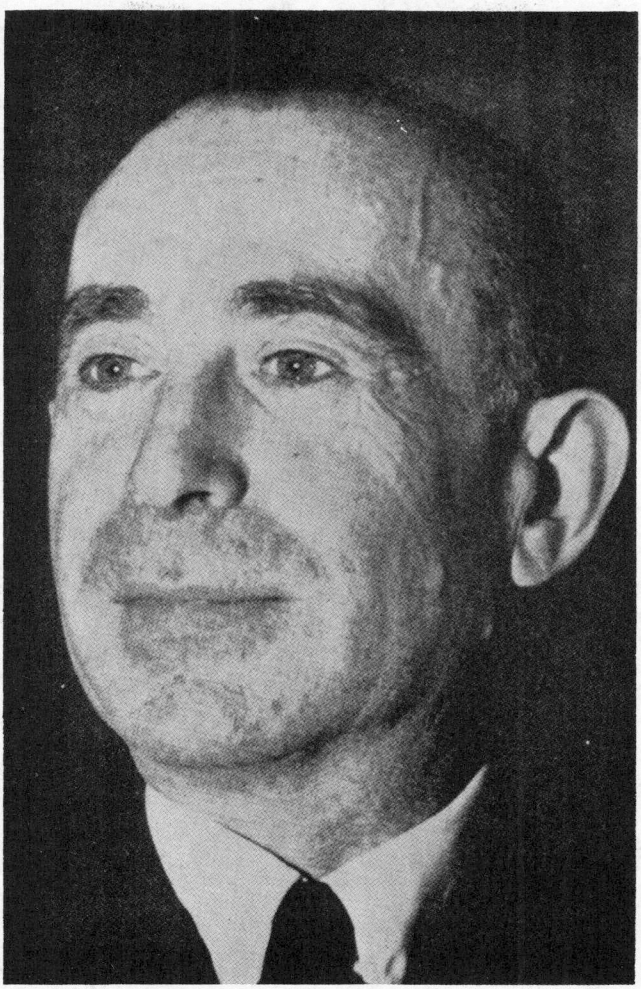

Manfred Sakel

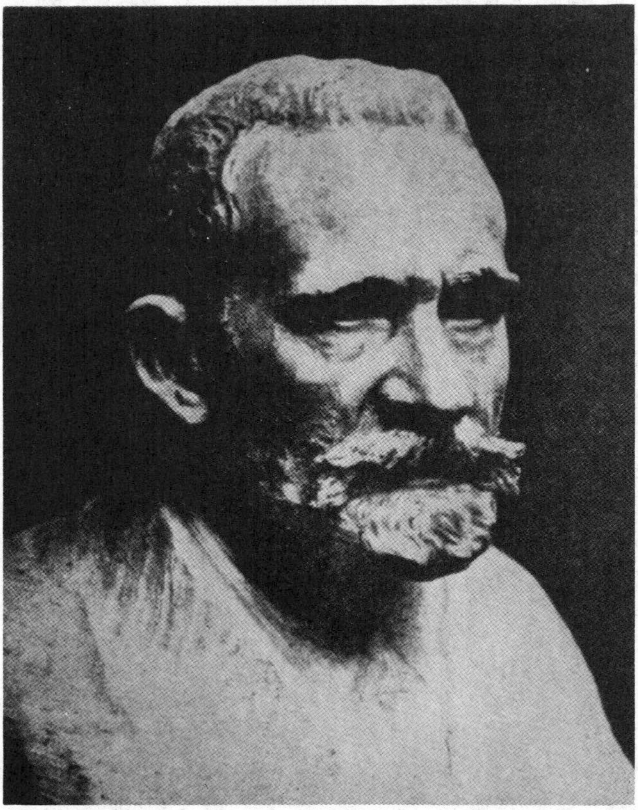

Emil Kraepelin

by his time: the nature of the soul, the origin and constitution of the temperaments, the result of humor combinations, and the senses; but there are elaborations on a more enlightened level and deviations from the ancient masters.

Vives' conception of memory is in advance of his age. He distinguishes between *recordatio*, which is an animal function, and *reminescentia*, which is peculiar to man. Partly this is the difference between mere learning and conscious recognition and recall gained through systematic mental search. Vives localizes memory in the occiput, and metaphorically refers to it as "the eye" which surveys the past. Preoccupation with the fluids in the brain is found in Vives, as in all ancient and medieval psychology. Whereas, Vives theorizes, impression is aided by a warm and moist brain, retention is favored by a firm and dry condition. Vives is strong on definitions and clear formulations and appears to be the first to have stated in precise terms the law of association. He observes, although with little justice, that the less important idea will lead to the more important, but not vice versa. He even vaguely adumbrates the law of conditioning. (When an animal enjoys something at the sounding of a tone, then when the tone is heard, it will expect the object it enjoyed previously.) His excursions into typology, based, of course, on the Galenian schema, are interesting in that he cites illustrations from life.

More on Vives will be said in the section dealing with medical psychology.

PHILIPP MELANCHTHON (1497-1560)— Preceptor of Germany

The coadjutor of Martin Luther, who had given him the theological slant, Philipp Melanchthon (which is the Greek for Schwarzerd, his real name) at the age of twenty-one was recommended by his uncle, Johann Reuchlin, chief of the Renaissance Humanists, to fill the chair in classics at the University of Wittenberg, where Luther taught.

Primarily a scholar, possibly as erudite as Erasmus, and even more versed in Greek than the great Dutchman, Melanchthon afterward became a theologian, but for whose skillful defenses of the new doctrines taught by Luther, Protestantism might have failed to take the almost insuperable hurdles which Luther could not have negotiated alone.

Frail in body and undistinguished in appearance, Melanchthon succeeded in commanding the respect of both the mighty and the lowly through his moderation, integrity, matchless Latin diction, untiring effort, and logical development of his discourses. It is not surprising that he was called the Preceptor of Germany; for, burdened though he was with teaching and reconciling the various forces that were at war with one another during this critical period, and with preparing the first code of Protestantism, he nevertheless found the time to write a psychological textbook, and to supervise as well as revise the educational system in Germany.

Even though he wrote, as was the custom of the

day, in Latin, he may be regarded as the first German psychologist; and it was he who first used the word "*psychologia*" in his lectures. Many previously had spoken about the soul, but none had thought of dignifying the material of their discourses with some substantival designation savoring of science. Psychology was simply a phase of physics.

Melanchthon laid no claim to originality. The very title of his work, *Commentarius de Anima,* which appeared in 1540, indicated that it was intended as a commentary on Aristotle's *De Anima,* which was generally garbled in translation due to the lack of Greek scholars. Thus Melanchthon, who was the world's chief authority on Greek, was the logical man to interpret the original, and elaborate on it in the light of contemporary knowledge.

Melanchthon's only rivals were his German colleague, Veit Amerbach, whose textbook is practically a Latin version of Aristotle's *De Anima,* and the Spaniard, Vives, who exercised a great influence in his day and later. Melanchthon's work appeared two years later than Vives' *De Anima et Vita,* and between 1540 and 1584 passed through twelve editions.

Vives, like his compatriot and younger contemporary, Huarte, was inclined to favor Galen as against Aristotle, but Melanchthon's analysis of certain concepts showed an independence of mind that was not common four hundred years ago. In his analysis of conscience, for example, he is not satisfied with the cognitive alone, as the etymology of the word would imply, but posits a "feeling" element, which Vives does not consider. ("*Manet etiam in corde vindex sclerum, horribilis dolor . . .*"). The affect is important, and not the idea.

In general, Melanchthon had an eye and ear for what had been despised among theoreticians. In his educational reforms, he rejected dogmatism. There was nothing of the stuffed shirt in him. If he admired Cicero, he nevertheless would not part with the sophisticate, Terence. It was because life meant more to him than cloister lucubrations that his *Commentary* had such a wide success.

It was not until three decades after his death that the word "*psychologia,*" which Melanchthon used only in one of his lectures, appeared as the title of a book: *Psychologia—Hoc Est de Hominis Perfectione* (*Psychology—That Is on the Perfecting of Man*), by the now completely forgotten Rudolf Goeckel.

GOCLENIUS

Goeckel (1547-1628), a Marburg professor of philosophy, will be recognized by students of formal logic as the formulator of the Goclenian Sorites. The word "*Psychologia*" in the title of his book was Greek, while the rest was in Latin. The work's popularity is attested by the fact that within seven years, it required three printings.

Goclenius, or Goeckel, who leaned toward Aristotle but was eclectic enough to side sometimes with Plato, was often extolled as the Marburg Plato, the Christian Aristotle, the "Light of Europe," and in other such hyperboles, but he was too steeped in scholastic issues to blaze a new path in philosophy. He could descant on such problems as whether an angel could at the same time occupy space in heaven and on our earth, whether the tongue was given us in order to speak or to taste, whether the primary purpose of the art of warfare is victory, etc. His psychological dichotomies, too, are sterile, e.g., dividing tears into cold and warm, thick and thin, sweet and bitter. For his time, however, there was something progressive in his aligning psychological with physiological processes, but theology was still to him, as to nearly all others in his century, the supreme tribunal which decided in matters of doubt. Philosophy was thus the handmaid of theology. His chief service lies in his logic; and the Goclenian sorites is a product of his dialectic preoccupation.

A few years later, Goeckel's follower, Otto Casmann, started the empirical trend by qualifying the material of his treatise as *Psychologia Anthropologica*. By narrowing its range, he was able to bypass the sterile scholasticism revolving around a rational psychology. It will be shown later why the profound Kant was pleased to call the psychology he taught, and which was afterward published, *Anthropologie*.

JUAN HUARTE (*c.* 1530-1589)—First Differential Psychologist, Pioneer of Testing Theory

Our histories of psychology seem to have neglected the man who, in 1575, through his *Examen de Ingenios* (*Probe of Minds*) put psychology, so to speak, on the map.

Huarte was a Spanish physician, probably of Basque origin who, unlike his colleagues who preceded and followed him, did not bother with speculations about the soul. He was interested in practical questions which bordered on biology and embryology but were essentially psychological in emphasis. We may put Huarte down as the man who suggested mental testing. The English translation of 1698 titles Huarte's book *The Tryal of Wits, Discovering the Great Differences of Wits Among Men and What Sort of Learning Suits Best With Each Genius.* From the title itself one gathers that the writer's purpose was to guide youth and advise parents on the aptitude of their children.

In his long dedicatory letter to King Philip, he comes right to the point:

> For considering how short and limited the wit of man is to one thing and no more, I have been always of opinion that no man could understand two arts perfectly well, without proving defective in one of them: and that accordingly none might err in the choice of that which was most agree-

> able to the bent of his natural inclination, there should be *Triers* appointed by the state, men of approved sagacity and knowledge, to search and sound the abilities of youth, and after due search, to oblige them to the study of that science their heads leaned most to, instead of abandoning them to their own choice.

In a most modern spirit, writing nearly four hundred years ago, the author astutely observes:

> All the ancient philosophers have found by experience, that where nature disposes not a man for knowledge, 'tis in vain for him to labor in the rules of the art. But not one of them has clearly and distinctly declared what that nature is, which renders a man fit for one, and unfit for another science, nor what difference of wit is observed among men, nor what arts and sciences are most suitable to each man in particular, nor by what marks they may be discerned, which is one of the greatest importance.

Without spreading his praise *ad nauseam,* as was customary in those days, Huarte asks the King to read the last chapter in order to discover what he might have excelled in, had he been born a commoner.

Why was it that this book became a best seller, meriting twenty-seven editions in Spanish alone, twenty-four in French, seven in Italian, five and, in addition, a long extract in English, three in Latin, one in Dutch, and two in German, one of them having the distinction of being made by no less a person than the dramatist, Lessing? A facsimile of the old English translation of this work has just come out. There are not many psychology books, even today, with millions of students throughout the world, which can lay claim to such interest. The first edition was gotten out by the author himself in fifteen hundred copies.

While it is true that Huarte took his substance from Aristotle, and to a greater degree from Galen, and, as was wont in those days, leaned heavily on verses from the Bible, he nevertheless plunges *in medias res* by examining the concept of intelligence (*ingenio,* from the Latin, *ingenium*) and investing the term with what we might today call "productive imagination."

The characteristics of intelligence are, according to him: (a) docility in learning from a master; (b) understanding and independence of judgment; and (c) inspiration without extravagance. The citations from Greek authors and the illustrations derived both from biography and history carry the reader along in a way that the barren verbiage of the day seldom achieved.

Huarte, to be sure, is preoccupied with all sorts of ancient hypotheses in regard to the humors, and makes much of the difference between the moist and the dry, the cold and the hot, taking it as an explain-all of the most incredible phenomena, such as the speech of *neonates,* the Latin discourses of insane people who had never known the language; but after we have discarded the husk, there remains a kernel of provocative thought. In the custom of dispensing interesting tidbits of information from the classics, he is not far behind Montaigne, but whereas the Frenchman simply makes observations, Huarte tries to reason and weigh conclusions.

Basing much of his thesis on the proportion of heat and moisture in the organism, he suggests curious differences between man and man, and between one nation and another. Since memory requires great moisture, the Germans excel in it, since they are full of it, but lacking the hot element, they are deficient in imagination. In accordance with Galen's observation that "those who dwell Northerly are defective in understanding, and those situated between the North and the torrid zone are most prudent," he puts Spain on a pedestal. If we can believe what he cites from Aristotle, then the Flemings, Germans, English, and French possess an intelligence reminiscent of drunkards, "for which reason they could not search into or know the nature of things." Huarte tells us the reason for this is the abundance of moisture which dilates the body and accounts for the larger stature and bulk of, for example, the Germans.

Despite his divagations and extravagations on the cold, moist seed which produces a girl and the hot, dry seed which produces a boy, and on the relation of food to intelligence, Huarte may be regarded as one of the enlightened men of his age, who inaugurated the study of differential psychology and foresaw the applications of intelligence testing.

The questions which Huarte undertakes to answer in the last chapter of his work are legion, and they deal mainly with the differences in man as a result of diverse conditions of copulation. Thus he asks why women of easy virtue do not easily miscarry, while respectable wives do on the slightest accident, why "bastards are generally personable, courageous and very discreet" and seeks his explanations in the relative force, moisture, and heat of the seed.

In other words, Huarte may also be taken as a pioneer in the field of eugenics, misinformed though he was in many respects—but let us note that he wrote his best-seller nearly four hundred years ago. Science has advanced a bit since. Parapsychologists may yet claim him as their own, for in one place in Chapter VII, he has this to say: "For there is a power and kind of nature which penetrates and predicts things to come, the force and character of which has never yet been explained by reason."

RENE DESCARTES (1596-1650)

Generally known as the father of modern philosophy and more famous for his dictum "*Cogito ergo sum*," which sounded the knell of dogmatism in philosophy, than for founding the branch of analytic geometry, he takes a prominent place in the history of psychology by virtue of (a) his analysis of the emotions (*Les Passions de l'Ame*); (b) his doctrine of interaction between body and soul; (c) his sharp division of man and animal, ascribing a soul to the former, while regarding the latter as an automaton without the power of thought; (d) the localization of the soul in the pineal gland; and (e) the rejection of the then prevailing belief of perception.

Descartes, like McDougall three hundred years later, thought that some psychic unity combined the images of both eyes into a single perception, and that that process was the function of the pineal gland. His analysis of joy and sorrow, as well as love and hatred, contains a tinge of psychosomatic doctrine.

THOMAS HOBBES (1588-1679)

Together with Francis Bacon, a friend who received far more recognition, Thomas Hobbes may be said to have elevated the tradition of Roger Bacon and Ockham, about whom they both knew little, to a school. Francis Bacon's concern with psychology appears only in a number of astute observations, scattered through his *Essays* and *Advancement of Learning,* and in his grasp of the principle of association. Otherwise, he is a methodologist and, in a minor sense, a metaphysician.

Hobbes, however, attempted to lay out a materialistic system which would include the realm of the mind as well; indeed, it would necessarily begin with it, for all phenomena have their origin there, and all knowledge is derived from the senses. He did not take any stock in innate ideas, but he went still farther and threw overboard all speculations that had come down from the Scholastic age and referred everything to the brain rather than the soul. Hence religious ideas were left severely alone or relegated to the province of faith. No wonder he acquired the reputation of being an atheist, and had many disputes with prelates.

In a sense, Hobbes must be regarded as the first behaviorist or operationist, for in his view, all our ideas come from our sensory experiences, and these are the results of stimuli *setting in operation the vital spirits.* Centuries before William James and Lange and Sergi, Hobbes had come to the conclusion that our emotions are the products of certain bodily movements. The soul is something tenuously corporeal —which is almost as good as saying "there is no soul." If thought to Watson was inner speech, imperceptible movement of the speech organs, then to Hobbes it consisted simply of addition and subtraction, as the origin of the term "calculate" would imply.

Hobbes's life work was a tripartite system of somatology, psychology, and political science. It was the last of the three which was involved in the short *De Cive,* and later the *Leviathan,* which can be regarded as a treatise on social psychology as well as politics. It also purports to offer an ethical code, but one based on self-interest, as the policy of "each one for himself," save for the need of protection against malefactors, can hardly come under the purview of ethics.

Hobbes's social psychology is akin to Machiavelli's. Indeed, Hobbes has been regarded as the chief philosophical theoretician of totalitarianism. In his day he extolled royalty, but in our age he would be strongly on the side of any dictatorship. In a perennial condition of *bellum omnium contra omnes* (war of all against all), the safest guarantee against chaos is absolute monarchy.

BARUCH (BENEDICT) SPINOZA (1632-1677)

The leading pantheist, and one of the foremost philosophers of all times, Spinoza brought into psychology the theory of psychophysical parallelism in place of Descartes's interactionism, and gave a close-knit formulation of the various emotions, both primary and derived, which is astounding in its modernity. Joy, sadness, and desire are the crucial emotions, which, with the adjuncture of ideas, yield a variety of additional emotions. Thus: "Hatred is sadness (pain) accompanied by the idea of an external cause." "Derision is joy arising from the fact that we imagine what we despise is present in what we hate."

Spinoza assumes that his deductive method carries conviction, but his truths are the result of his intuitive insights. It is in the notes and the scholia that his great mind reveals itself. The geometrical method to Spinoza, some three hundred years ago, was equivalent to the experimental method of today.

There is a great deal in Spinoza that has not been adequately evaluated. Dogmatic—or rather, as he would deem it, rigid—in method, he is most critical in his observations. In one of his enlightening notes (*Ethics* II, 17) he alludes to his empirical approach. "Nor do I think that I have wandered far from the truth, since all the postulates I have assumed scarcely contain anything that is not borne out by experience."

Spinoza foreshadowed Hume when he declared in a corollary: "For the mind knows not itself save insofar as it perceives ideas of modifications of the body. But it does not perceive its body save through the ideas of modifications, through which also it only perceives external bodies." He points out the conflict which arises from loving another who does not reciprocate, a conflict arising from the pleasure involved in love and the pain attached to hate. He emphasizes individual differences in the proposition (*Ethics* III, 57): "Any emotion of every individual differs from the emotion of another only insofar as the constitution of the one differs from that of the other." Reason is the criterion in ethics as well as in life. Mental hygiene is an affiliate of reason; and the biological standpoint is uppermost in Spinoza's system.

Endowed with a most serene temperament, he was subjected to persecution, turmoil, and threats. There can be no doubt that Spinoza would have become a beacon in psychology had he not come to an untimely death, in his forties, worn out by the manual labor of grinding lenses by day and intense mental concentration at night, in addition to being harrowed, after his excommunication by the rabbis, by both Jewish fanatics and Christian bigots.

JOHN LOCKE (1632-1704)

A special student in medicine without benefit of a degree, Locke, like Goethe, Leibniz, and Hobbes, served as adviser, supervisor, and tutor. He was fortunate to be connected with the Shaftesbury family in such capacity, and was influential in bringing about liberal reforms. It was said that he had a hand in drafting the charter of the Carolinas.

Locke's philosophical propensities developed late, but when his *Essay Concerning Human Understanding* appeared, he was destined to become the first of a new dynasty, which is not altogether defunct today—the first of the three patriarchs in British empiricism. Without Locke, there might never have been either Berkeley or Hume. The subject of *substance,* whether material or spiritual, was discarded in his system, which set out to present a thorough analysis of *ideas,* in a very broad sense. He is averse to all nativism. At birth, the mind is a *tabula rasa,* but experiences keep accumulating in the form of sensations and perceptions, which are compounds of sensation and affection. He indulges in long discussions of primary and secondary qualities, of various kinds of ideas and their origin, of words, of knowledge, and of opinion. He was the first to coin the phrase "association of ideas."

Locke's success (in English alone there must have been close to a hundred editions to date of the *Essay*) was due largely to his publicistic style. His illustrations are copious and often quaint but effective. Without mentioning Hobbes, he subtly attacks the notion that movement can produce thought. His arguments for the existence of God are more original and discursive than those of his predecessors, and if one grants the premises, his reasoning is cogent, but that part of his *Essay* does not fall under the psychological rubric. The *Essay* as a whole, however, may be regarded as a textbook in psychology, free of all scholastic and dogmatic appurtenances.

GEORGE BERKELEY (1685-1753)

If John Locke, the Englishman, attacked the dragon of metaphysics with his critical spear, and sought to reinstate the primary qualities of objects as objective and real, Bishop Berkeley, the Irishman, while availing himself of the method, tore down the primary qualities (like hardness) as well as the secondary (like color), and argued that a wall was no more real than the feeling of agreeableness which warmth gave, and that therefore there was nothing objective and independently real in the world *except the mind.*

In other words, Berkeley turned Locke's psychology inside out, and became the pillar of idealism. True, Samuel Johnson gave the wall a vehement kick to prove the absurdity of Berkeley's notion, but to Berkeley the kick was immaterial, and the bricks were still just a matter of sight and touch or resistance—in a word, ideas and nothing more. In his dialogues, he argued that sounds which are not heard do not exist. ("And can any sensation exist without the mind? How then can sound, being a sensation, exist in the air if by the air you mean a senseless substance existing without the mind?") If sound is due to motion in the air then sound should be felt or seen but never heard.

Just as Descartes is remembered by his slogan "*Cogito ergo sum,*" so Berkeley's "*Esse est percipi*" ("To be is to be perceived") has become a watchword in later idealism. What is not perceived does not exist, but since such a situation would divest the world of its existence, Berkeley finds the solution in God. We are all ideas in the mind of God. Thus Berkeley sidetracked the paraphernalia of physics, of which in earlier years psychology was a part (at Harvard University, for about a century, psychology was a department of physics called pneumatology) and turned the tables, so that psychology included all of physics in order to lead up to the *prima causa,* in metaphysics, and to the font of theology.

Berkeley's chief contribution to psychology was his new theory of vision, on genetic or empirical principles. Locke had already taught that a blind person who knew the difference between cubes and spheres through touch could not, on receiving sight, tell which was which. This was one form of the refutation of innate ideas. Now Berkeley went the whole hog and brought out some original notions. "We never see and feel one and the same object," he tells us. "That which is seen is one thing and that which is felt is another." We can sense how he paved the way—to his own abhorrence had he realized it—to Hume's absolute sensationalism. Modern theories of space perception are in line with Berkeley's observations on clues which we interpret, which he called "suggestions." We see lights and colors suggesting a tree, and perceive the suggestion of resistance or solidity because of our past experience of resistance, a purely subjective quality. Thus we have the paradox that this time it was not the intellectualist who brought idealism to the fore but an out-and-out empiricist.

DAVID HUME (1711-1776)

The greatest of the British trio who consolidated empiricism, Hume, the Scotsman, went the Irishman, Berkeley, one better. Agreeing that there is no real proof of the existence of objects, he applied the same arguments to the self and made the famous statement in the penetrating book which he wrote at the age of twenty-seven, that whenever he contemplates the self he stumbles upon nothing but sense impressions. Thus not only did he throw the soul out of the window, but even the "self," "ego," or "I" became a mere bundle of sensations. In other words, he completed the circuit which Locke broke and by making a philosophical somersault, he turned a corner in philosophy. The great Kant found it imperative to devise means for saving the world from the devastation which Hume's skepticism would have brought about.

Hume's youthful lucubration was so thoroughgoing in its trenchant probing that his influence is felt to this day, not only in philosophy but in physical theory as well. His conclusions, however, were arrived at through psychological considerations. With a relentless logic he pursues his inquiry into the origin of ideas, dividing them into ideas proper and impressions, which latter would correspond to our sensations, perceptions, and emotions—in other words, any mental experience called forth by an external stimulus.

Perhaps Hume's greatest feat was his telling attack on the principle of causality. The chief argument of realists was that our sense impressions point to causes which must be outside us. The idealist, on the other hand, doubting the material existence of objects when they are not perceived, took God for their sponsor, since He perceives everything at all times. Hume will not accept that as a guarantee, and therefore can be sure only of his sense impressions—thus giving rise to the system of phenomenalism. Since one urges, however, that the sense impression must have a cause, he goes to the very root of this universally accepted truth and demolishes it by arguing that causality is nothing but a sort of illusion, arising out of the smooth transition from one idea to another. We see two things following one another so often that we read into it some mysterious power or relationship, but in reality the real mystery lies in the constant, although not necessary, association of ideas. Hume regarded this bond as a law corresponding to Newton's law of gravitation; and although he had no idea of the neural basis of association, he recognized only three forms of connection among ideas, namely, resemblance, contiguity in place and time, and causality. These, of course, are only ideas, relations, or associations, and not necessarily substantial.

Hume's life is as odd as his philosophy, which he was already projecting as an undergraduate at college. Like Hobbes and Locke, he held no academic post, but served as a minor attaché in foreign service or as a librarian. Disgusted because his "juvenile" book, as he called it, fell stillborn from the press, he turned to history and became more widely known as a historian than as a philosopher.

His autobiographical sketch is a masterpiece of objectivity and his equanimity approaching death at the age of sixty-five, probably of cancer, is characteristic of the man and his temper. "I consider," he writes, "that a man of 65, by dying cuts off only a few years of infirmities." He tells us that "I possess the same ardor as ever in study, and the same gayety in company."

Hume's name will continue to shine in the firmament of philosophy and psychology, despite his negative rather than positive achievements, and his straying from the philosophical arena.

GOTTFRIED WILHELM LEIBNIZ (1646-1716)

A full-fledged scholar and thinker at the age of twenty, Leibniz shone equally in mathematics (sharing the honors, at least in Germany, with Newton in the discovery of infinitesimal calculus), diplomacy, and philosophy. Trained for the legal profession, he became financial adviser, administrator, and librarian in the employ of German nobility, a situation which afforded him opportunities for travel and leisure. He was instrumental in the founding of the Berlin Academy of the Sciences, serving as its first president.

Unlike Spinoza, Leibniz was fundamentally a metaphysician, a philosophical trouble-shooter, and dogmatist par excellence. He may be looked upon as the antipode of Spinoza, whom he met and whose *Ethics* he read in manuscript with a view to refuting it. Encyclopedic in his range of knowledge, he nevertheless took little interest in the physiological or biological, and concentrated on the ingenious. His doctrine of monads and pre-established harmony outside of our domain need not be explained here. Instead of the soul-atom, which he called the monad, he might have directed his attention, microcentric as he was, upon the nerve cell, but that was reserved for someone else. Leibniz did not even bother with the relation of body and mind, as did Descartes and Spinoza. He found a ready formula in the principle of pre-established harmony, operating, naturally, by the grace of God; and that was that.

Leibniz's entrance into the controversy between

the nativists and the empiricists did take him into the midst of psychological theorizing. Hobbes had already started the ball of empiricism rolling, and Locke was to fight out the issue against innate ideas to the bitter end, but Leibniz plunged into the fray full tilt, and to Locke's insistence on the old dictum, "There is nothing in the intellect which had not previously come to the senses," Leibniz shot out a triumphant "except the intellect itself." Incidentally, it has been stated by a number of historians of psychology that Leibniz's refutation of Locke's *Essay* was never published, since Locke died just as it was being completed, but the rebuttal is to be found in the *Nouveaux Essais,* published posthumously.

Perhaps Leibniz's chief contribution to psychology was his claim that there were certain perceptions below the threshold of awareness, which he called "*petites perceptions,*" while the conscious perceptions which we talk about he designated "apperceptions." He thus introduced the concept of the subconscious (not Freud's unconscious) centuries ago. It was Leibniz's understanding that the roar of the sea which we hear is only an accumulation of the singly imperceptible wave sounds.

CONDILLAC (1715-1780)

French psychology did not produce the giants we find in Germany. After Descartes, there was no single outstanding name until we come to Condillac, who showed at least a modicum of originality in his *Traité des Sensations* (1754), which was superior in scope and conception to his earlier work, *Sur les Connaissances Humaines.*

It was through a woman follower that Condillac received the first impetus to reconsider his differences with Locke, and he ended up by going Locke one better, without being in the least disturbed over the fact that as an *abbé,* he was taking a radical stand when he maintained that the mind consists of nothing but sensations and its derivatives.

As Pavlov experimented with a dog in order to establish his system of reflexology, Condillac, with the aid of his lady pupil, engaged in shadow experimentation on a statue, which they imagined could explain the successive unfolding of its senses and higher mental functions. Which is the first sense to develop? Condillac believed it is smell. Now as different objects are smelled, a rose, turpentine, onions, etc., one will stand out more vividly than the other. Thus we have *attention,* which selects the particular odor.

The next sense to emerge is touch, then sight. Every sensation occurs together with the quality of agreeableness or disagreeableness, providing the basis of our *feelings.* Memory comes when previous impressions have been revived. Sensations are compared, and therefore we acquire *judgment.* Judgment and memory, when they become routine from sheer frequency, *yield habit.* As for emotions, they all revolve around the feelings, which are attributes of sensations. Thus, when some new sensation strikes the statue, *astonishment* may result, or *fear* or *anger.* Will is the culmination of accumulated desires, and is last to form.

This, like later behaviorism in the United States, which also introduced (Singer) a mechanical sweetheart, sounds so simple and matter-of-fact that many of the easygoing French thinkers, particularly the nascent Encyclopedists, gobbled it up, fancying that in so doing they had become enlightened. Condillac was an empiricist and affected French psychology for many decades, until Maine de Biran made an effort to bring into the picture the *will.* In place of Descartes's "*Cogito ergo sum,*" his motto became "*Je veux donc je suis*" ("I will, therefore I am"). He would thus be aligned with the contemporary hormic school, of which McDougall was the leading representative.

In Bonnet (1720-1793), a Swiss naturalist, Condillac had an able follower, who was a field worker, sedulously observing his insects. He was not satisfied with mere enumerations and derivations, but, interested in some of the English philosophical writers, he was eager to anchor the psychological facts to a physiological base; and he saw in vibrations which are conveyed along the nerves to the brain the actual process which causes sensation. Whether he knew of Tetens and his oscillatory doctrine of brain action, to explain memory, for instance, is doubtful, but probably the vibratory character of sound conduction was suggestive in both instances.

THE FIRST PSYCHOLOGICAL JOURNAL*

CARL PHILIP MORITZ

Before leaving Germany, it behooves us to become acquainted with one of the most remarkable men of the century, who, although neither a psychologist nor a medical man, did much to advance our knowledge of human nature. This was Carl Philipp Moritz (1756-1793).

Moritz was a very brilliant meteor, whose light was extinguished at the age of thirty-six, after a ceaseless struggle against poverty, migraine, tuberculosis, and depressive moods which alienated a number of his friends, but in the short span which was allowed him, he was able to accomplish what has fallen to the lot of very few even of the more gifted.

Born into a Quietist family, he was introduced by his stepfather to the mysticism of the group, part of whose ritual was to spend a definite period in abstract meditation, in a sort of contentless silence. This must have been the source of his later program of analytic introspection. One might even coin the word "autoscopy" (looking into oneself) or "psychoscopy," something different from the laboratory method of introspection.

A wretched childhood, during which he made an attempt at suicide, is reflected in the first psychological novel to be written—*Anton Reiser*—an autobiography which served to turn the attention of educators to the problems of children. With a wealth of detail and fine discernment, the twenty-four-year-old author dwells on the inner life of the sensitive pre-adolescent. His later novel, *Andreas Hartknopf,* deals with the conflicts of the theological student.

Moritz was scarcely ten years old when his stepfather apprenticed him to a capmaker. However, some citizens in the community learned about the youngster's capabilities and arranged to have him sent to high school, where he showed great proficiency. He was training for the ministry but a series of circumstances intervened, and he becomes a bohemian, associating with questionable companions; and between acquiring books, which he devoured almost as a surrogate for the food he lacked, and preparing for a stage career, he spent much of his energy and substance in an agitated sentimentality which made him the butt of his associates, as he wavered between the theater and the church. In addition, he took on a teaching post, but in 1780, at the age of only twenty-four, he became co-rector.

About two years later, he journeyed to England, and explored the southern part on foot, giving us a most interesting account of the places, the inns, the customs and manners of the people, particularly the innkeepers and their help, whom he reviles in unmistakable terms, mentioning, however, that his arrival on foot as well as his garb likely made a poor impression. When he once asked a fellow traveler why the English, who were so enterprising, did not now and then, just to see life and nature from every angle, travel on foot instead of undergoing the discomfort of coach transportation, the reply was, "We are too rich, too lazy, and too proud"—in which he concurred, regarding the English as a race of snobs.

On returning to Berlin, he was appointed professor in a Gymnasium (a sort of junior college) and here he met the famous Moses Mendelssohn and noted Marcus Herz, and later the extraordinary Solomon Maimon—all three Jews who co-operated with Moritz to found the *Magazin zur Erfahrungsseelenkunde.*

One of the strange prodigies in the history of modern philosophy, Maimon subsequently became co-editor of the journal.

The *Magazin* was, in a sense, a protest against the theoretical and hair-splitting discussions of the essence of psychology. It stressed the empirical, as may be gathered from the word "*Erfahrung*." There were many articles on child psychology, delinquency, mental illness, defective children, linguistic psychology, and even what is now called extrasensory perception. The meat of the journal consisted of descriptions of cases and stimulating suggestions. Moritz did not by-pass methodological problems. He merely took a practical stand, and advocated analytical introspection as the staple of psychology. He would place psychology on a footing with organic medicine, seeking to establish a physiology of the soul or mind, and to start with the case as in medicine, working up to the principle, and not the other way around. He even speaks of psychic dietetics, in the form of ideas which each individual should be able to find as most suitable to his own mental constitution.

It may be surmised that Moritz did not fully realize his program. His was too desultory a mind to plumb problems systematically. He was no Kant nor Tetens to examine the foundations and proceed step by step in keeping with the postulates of a scientific methodology. But his intuitive flashes provoked thought, and his recourse to everyday events, or at least documentary instances, although not truly verified, furthered psychological interest and tended to pull psychology away from its metaphysical domination; and his insights were not to be waved aside.

Constituted as he was, a man of intense feelings, he did not care much for intellectualistic solutions. The affections loomed large in his quasi-system; and activity, he felt, was a necessary outlet. The *will* is interpreted in somewhat Spinozistic terms—namely, that the dwelling on an idea, whether good or bad, for any length of time, will lead to its execution—a modern view.

Moritz took leave of absence to travel through Italy, and when he returned after two years, he deplored the direction that the *Magazin's* acting editor, Pockels, had taken. Despite his newly won professorship at the Academy of Art in Berlin, and his other literary labors, he continued to edit the *Magazin,* this time with Maimon, although it is difficult to imagine how these two cantankerous natures could have worked together on such a project. With the death of Moritz, in his early prime, the *Magazin* ceased publication.

Not counting the *Magazin,* Moritz, in the dozen productive years vouchsafed him, wracked with pain and mental anguish, because of his supersensitiveness and excessive ambition in different areas, produced more than twenty volumes, embracing subjects such as psycho linguistics, prosody, travel, two novels, plastic imitation in aesthetics, mythology (nine editions), logic for children (as he supposed), essays and epigrams, a grammatical dictionary of German, pedagogy and psychology.

Goethe, Wilhelm von Humboldt, and even Schiller, whom he had previously deprecated to the extent of stating that it was with loathing that he picked up a Schiller play, thought highly of his intellect, Goethe saying that *Anton Reiser* was a mirror of his own youthful mind.

THOMAS BROWN (1778-1820)

Although Thomas Brown was not the patriarch of the Scottish Common Sense School (that honor was reserved for Thomas Reid, of St. Andrews and later of Glasgow University), and did not possess the originality of the youngest of that group, Sir William Hamilton, Brown was chiefly a psychologist, and his *Lectures on the Philosophy of the Human Mind,* published posthumously, is a combination textbook and treatise, containing over half a million words. Even if we disregard the last two hundred pages, devoted to ethics and metaphysics, we still have the equivalent of a thousand-page modern textbook, given over to a full and penetrating analysis of such topics as sensation, perception, suggestion, desire, emotion, disposition, etc. Much of Brown's presentation is taken up with mild polemics, particularly against Reid, whom he does not credit with having refuted Hume, or with having gone further than Locke in his theories.

Brown was conversant with not only British but also French philosophy, and to a less extent with German works. Having a literary bent of mind, he interspersed his well-written lectures with verse, sometimes in Latin, which added to the gracefulness of his style. Indeed, it was said he preferred poetry to philosophy, but his own verse received little recognition, possibly because he was ahead of his time in shunning the ordinary and indulging in less accessible imagery; and since philosophers do not welcome a division of talents, his academic activities were somewhat depreciated.

One of his advantages over his colleagues, although they would scarcely have admitted it, was his training in medicine. Hence he did not refer as frequently as they to "our gracious Creator," but would introduce the role of "Nature" in his explanations. His greatest asset is his use of copious illustrations from all walks of life.

The chief appeal of the Scottish School was to the activity of the mind. English empiricism was regarded as too mechanical; and thus association was thought to be beneath notice in the explication of mental phenomena. The term "intuition" had been a sort of trade-mark of the school, particularly in ethics, where the moral obligation is perceived by the average person, or as Brown puts it, "Persons acting in a certain manner, excite in us a feeling of approval; persons acting in a manner opposite to this [excite a feeling] . . . of an opposite kind." In this way, ethics is anchored to psychological states—feelings of approval and disapproval.

Since association was a term not in good repute among the "Common Sense" philosophers, other concepts were brought in. Reid made a great deal of "perception," while Brown made "suggestion" the cornerstone in his system. He does not deny that there are occasions on which simple similarity or contiguity in place or time are enough to produce a similar mental impression, but in most cases, he believes that some portion in a complex whole *suggests* another whole. In other words, there has been an activity which does not occur in a process like association. Herein, he reveals a leaning to the principle of Gestalt psychology. Similarly, Hamilton introduced the notion of *redintegration,* according to which a single element in a complex will reintroduce a former complex. In other words, the mental machinery operates less simply and more elaborately than associationism would imply.

Brown, who was only forty-two when he died, made another dent in the development of psychology; for he was the first to describe in detail the muscular sense, in a chapter entitled "Of the Feelings Usually Ascribed to the Sense of Touch." "The feeling of resistance," we read, "is, I conceive, to be ascribed not to our organ of touch but to our muscular frame," and in another place, "What is the feeling of fatigue, e.g., but a muscular feeling, that is to say, a feeling of which our muscles are as truly the organ as our eye or ear is the organ of sight or hearing." When we consider that these statements were made about 150 years ago, Brown's psychological insight must be acknowledged.

The Scottish thinkers, unlike the English, as Thomas Buckle had already observed in his stupendous work on English civilization, were metaphysicians. Their reasoning was deductive, while that of the English was inductive. Hume's empiricism, despite his Scottish ancestry, was ascribed by Buckle to his English environment.

While it is true that the Scottish School has not left an indelible impress on the course of psychology, it must not be forgotten that until the advent of William James, Harvard was dominated by the doctrines of Reid, Dugald Stewart and Brown, while Princeton was wholly under the sway of the Common Sense School until Baldwin started the laboratory there. Indeed, Baldwin may be said to have been a sprig of the same heather. William McDougall's philosophical outlook, which colored his psychology and his analysis of the emotions to a large extent, reflects his affiliation with the Scots.

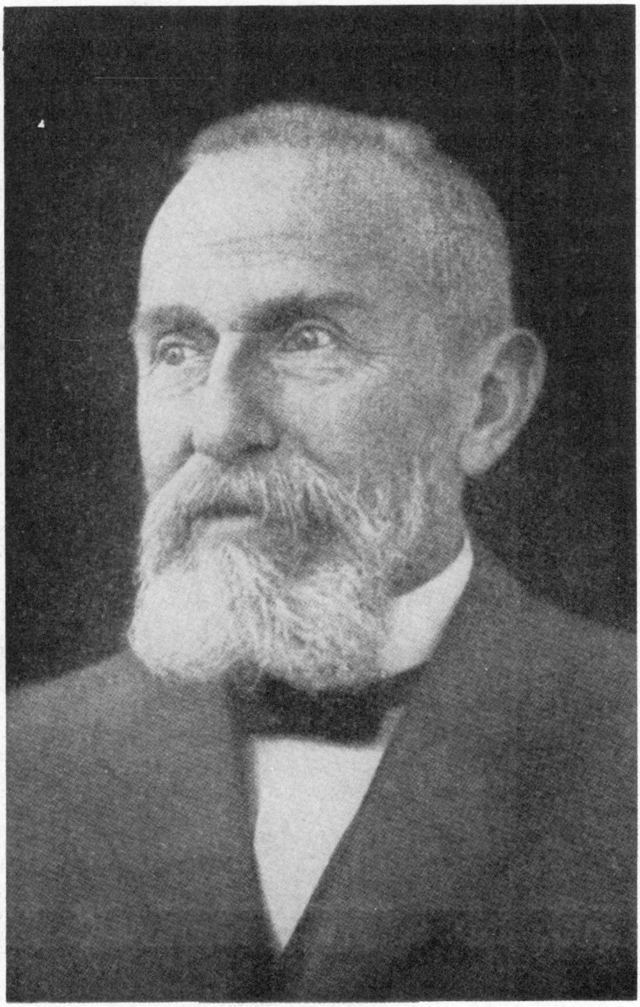

Eugen Bleuler

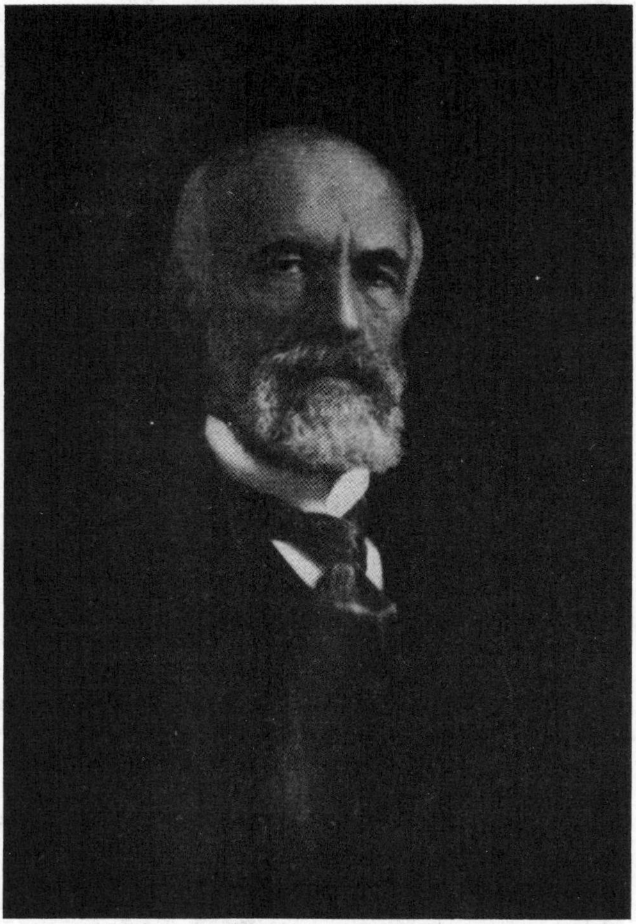

G. Stanley Hall

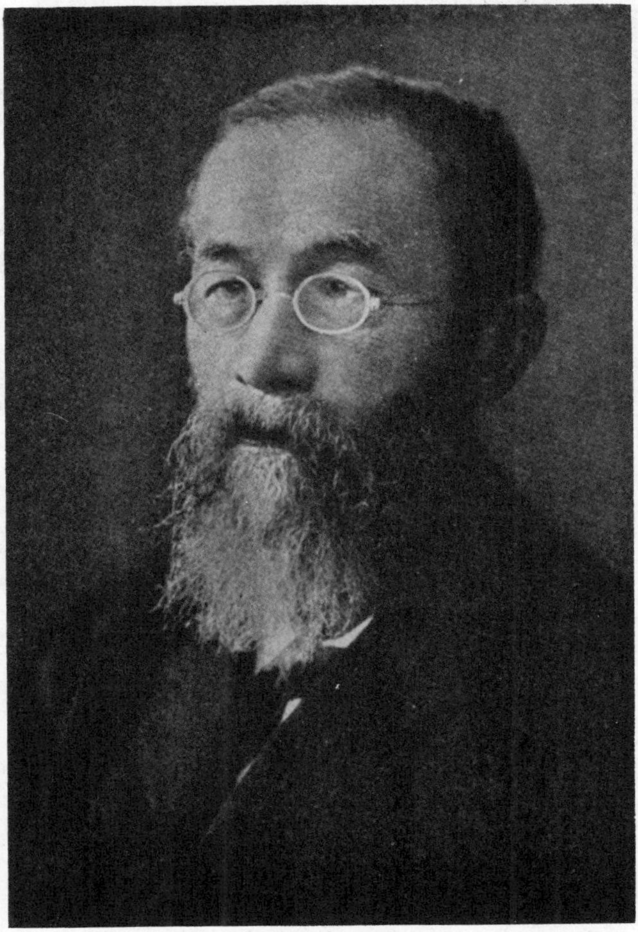

Wilhelm Wundt

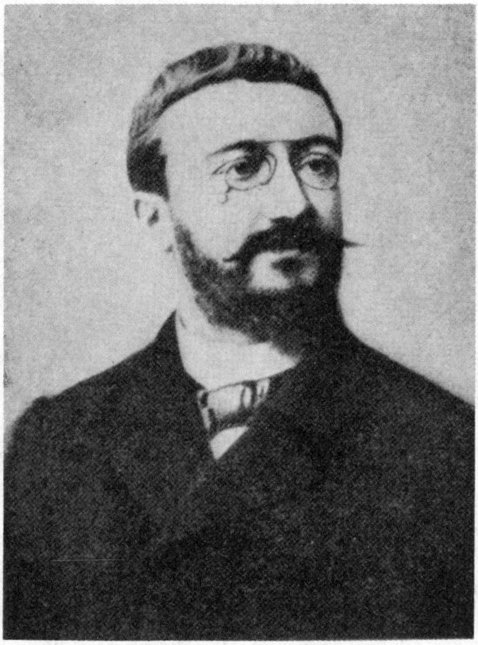

Alfred Binet

J. NICOLAS TETENS (1736-1807) and IMMANUEL KANT (1724-1804) Thresh Out Deep Issues

Tetens, contemporary of Kant, whose fame as a philosopher proved detrimental to the reputation of one who outshone him in psychology, may be regarded as the first German psychologist on a large scale. Just as Kant had a bit of Scots in him, Tetens was tinged with a Danish outlook. (Rostock was at one time in Danish territory and later Tetens both studied and taught at the University of Copenhagen, ending up virtually as finance minister of Denmark.) Tetens was not the profound philosopher that Kant is, but he was an authority in physics and mathematics, and, therefore, a scientist of a high order. His style is hardly less cumbersome than Kant's, but his subject-matter, being less metaphysical, makes his *Philosophical Essay on Human Nature* (1777) a bit more viable, especially as it is replete with homely illustrations and ingenious analogies.

Kant, apparently, considered psychology without status since it possessed neither the fundamental significance of epistemology and metaphysics nor the practical urgency of ethics; nor did it come under the heading of science, inasmuch as it did not permit of *quantification,* which to Kant was the chief criterion of a science, so that he did not even dignify chemistry with this designation. Tetens, on the other hand, forewent diving into the depths of philosophy, to present us with a closely reasoned analysis of mental states and a formulation of problems which must appear remarkable even today. His major treatise consists of at least half a million words, not to mention minor essays on such topics as the psychology of language, climate and character, and kindred questions.

In all that Tetens wrote, there is evidence of an extraordinarily critical mind, a mind that suggests rather than affirms, questions and ponders, and yet comes out with flashes which must have been too bright for the eyes of his colleagues.

Tetens was systematic. His table of contents is analytic, and one is made aware of his steps. It would take too much space to enumerate all his conclusions, but some of them are as follows:

The independence and role of the feelings, a conclusion which brings him closer to the modern dynamic position than to the psychologists of his day.

He accepted introspection as a method, despite the arguments which Comte, and a century later the behaviorists, advanced against it. Tetens admitted that it is next to impossible to observe and at the same time observe the observing process, but he maintained that what we are actually observing is the reflection of the *direct observance as it appears to an immediate memory.*

Tetens also studied the problems of memory. How do we retain ideas? When he speaks of material ideas, he means brain processes. He conjectures that the brain is composed of a substance which allows of some slow oscillation of its fibers (possibly molecules, if he had thought in microscopic terms), so that memory may be a lasting echo. He does not lose sight of difficulties with this theory, such as change of texture with age, but at any rate, the very questions he brings up are of considerable account.

Tetens, the physical scientist, applied the laws of chemistry to the promotion of ideas and tells us (Vol. I, p. 138) that one is hard put to find modes of combination and dissolution in the chemical sphere which are not paralleled in the mental realm. Three laws of ideational formation (and dissolution) are drawn up, but he is not to be interpreted as a forerunner of the mental chemistry school of James and Stuart Mill, but rather as a forerunner of Gestalt psychology.

William James has been credited with bringing out the function of relational states which had been neglected to the advantage of substantive states, but here is a passage from Tetens which, written before 1777, gives food for thought in this connection. "An object lies close to another, yet stands apart. There is a symmetry and order to a building, a machine, etc. What are the *co-real relations* here? What is proximity? Distance? Contact? Apartness? . . . What is the objective and *absolute* in the forementioned relations of position and order, and wherein lies the *relative*, which only the understanding interposes?" (Vol. I, p. 277)

Tetens, though Kant's junior by a dozen years, mentions his great contemporary but rarely. Instead he refers to the names of Bonnet, Hartley, Search quite often. We must remember that Kant began to teach psychology, or anthropology, as he called it, late in life, and his book *Anthropology in Its Pragmatic Aspect* came out in his late seventies. It is not anthropology, as we understand it today, but empirical psychology, as distinguished from rational psychology, extended so as to go beyond the individual.

Kant's Strictures Against Psychology

Kant came to psychology panoplied as a knight of metaphysics. He had already, in his *Critique of Pure Reason,* dealt a death blow to the soul as a substance, and treated the self as a logical process (*synthetic unity of apperception*) which presumably must be physiologically grounded. Rational psychology, up to

Kant, revolved around the soul, but to Kant the soul is only a postulate of practical reason, in the interests of ethics and religion. Rational psychology dealt with this ego, this thinking self, in a strictly logical and a priori fashion, pitting proposition against proposition in order to gain a valid conclusion, but nothing empirical must enter in, or else the whole method will be invalidated by combining what cannot be combined.

Rational psychology considers the nature of fundamentals from the point of view of delimiting concepts, and is therefore a form of discipline rather than a body of facts. Empirical psychology, on the other hand, deals with observations on the mental experiences of the individual, and because these are subjective, the body of data cannot come under the head of science, but constitutes a series of observations and opinions. If anything, rational psychology is more of a science, because it manipulates concepts, as in mathematics or logic, but it is of mighty small compass; for it occupies itself only with the self as a thinker, its phases and gradations, its differentiation from other concepts (matter, space, time). Empirical psychology covers all sensation, emotion, perception, ideas, etc., but they can only be registered. There is no a priori principle involved, hence *we cannot find any causal relationship or predict events.*

Kant's anthropology is the psychology of the individual considered in relation to the whole. In other words, social behavior, customs, and folkways come in for consideration. Although Kant never left the town of Königsberg, he was quite at home in political geography and ethnic lore, and his *Anthropologie* is the most entertaining of his works, yet curiously enough it is one of the very few books of his not to have been translated into English. The reason, no doubt, is that it is regarded as much inferior to his greater works, bespeaking an indifferent attitude, as when a symphony conductor of rigid standards stoops to offer a pops concert.

Kant, nevertheless, anticipated much of the later criticism of introspection. He appears to have adhered to a psychophysical parallelism more than Tetens, who felt that the "I" had no neural counterpart, and his influence has penetrated psychology through various channels—e.g., through his conviction that space and time are original intuitions of the mind, he gave the first impetus to nativistic theories in perception.

As regards the distinction between the rational and empirical phases, Kant had already found the distinction in his older contemporary, Christian Wolff, a follower of Leibniz, who applied the doctrine of monads to the relation of body and soul, but Kant with his over-all critical method brought the matter to a more definitive conclusion.

J. FRIEDRICH HERBART (1776-1841)— First Dynamic Psychologist

Herbart, the successor of Kant at the University of Königsberg, is known mainly for his doctrine of apperception, but he achieved a great deal more in psychology, and particularly in applied education. An outgoing personality, who took a deep interest in the community, and refused to spend his time building up a metaphysical system, he was instrumental in improving the German school system. In that respect, he did not fall into the category of the average German professor of philosophy. Perhaps his coming from around Bremen, a seaport, had something to do with his more cosmopolitan tendency, which also expressed itself in marriage to an English girl.

Herbart started where Kant left off, so far as psychology was concerned. He first made short shrift of the faculties. The term was, if not a misnomer, at least nondescript. He was interested in processes, in action. In one sense, he could be regarded as a sympathizer of the Lockean school of ideas, but while Locke and his successors were content with a phenomenological treatment of ideas, i.e., just the awareness, Herbart went deeper and spoke of the *force* inherent in each idea. Therein lies his greatness as a pioneer, for we may think of him as the first dynamic psychologist.

Starting with a metaphysical concept "Real," which is the unit of existence, reminiscent of Leibniz's "monad" and perhaps also of our nuclear particles, he proceeds to erect an imposing structure. The interrelation of ideas is due to the clash of these Reals or force centers, which are either positively or negatively charged. Herbart even uses the term "complex," although not with the Freudian connotation. Similarly he makes much of ideas dropping below the threshold of consciousness and, though the individual is not aware of it, exerting some influence on what goes on in consciousness. Since the force behind the idea is real, it does not, theoretically, ever disappear. This is of a piece with the Freudian conception of mental energy, which is conserved as a constant, and is disturbed by conflicts. One should not conclude, however, that Herbart had any notion of psychoanalysis, though he certainly thought in terms of dynamic psychology.

In his quasi-Leibnizian metaphysics, Herbart believes the soul to be a Real, situated in the brain, unknowable in its ultimate nature, but only as it is activated by stimuli.

On the empirical side, Herbart tried to cope with the very difficulty which caused Kant to deny to psychology any scientific status; for he set out to treat the ideational processes mathematically, thinking up formulae in the matter of inhibition and facilitation, attraction and repulsion. Despite the fact that the whole calculus was highly conjectural, we see nevertheless that Herbart was perhaps the first to conceive the notion of working with a model; and while C. L. Hull, in our own time, had a more scientific apparatus and more rigorous standards for his behavior schemes, the method was essentially the same, and the results perhaps not less problematic.

Herbart's influence on the course of education and psychology was immense, and his popularity as a lecturer was so great that there was scarcely a hall large enough at the University to accommodate the students. It was through his enthusiasm, his practicality, and public-spiritedness that he acquired pupils and followers who transmitted his views and methods to their pupils, until his ideas took hold even in the United States, with teacher seminars and training colleges springing up in various places. Many were the Herbartian societies founded in various parts of Europe and America. The American one alone numbered two thousand members. It is not generally known that the parent of the influential National Society for the Study of Education, with its thousands of members, was once called the National Herbart Society, thus pointing to Herbart as the patron saint of all teachers.

The thirty-five letters constituting *The Application of Psychology to the Science of Education* are a model of clarity and argumentation, on the basis of experience. Much of what he sets forth in these letters addressed to a former pupil and friend of long standing (F. K. Griepenkerl) is still valid.

Herbart's illustrations in the matter of inhibition and facilitation are, except for the actual drawings, topological in character, and they can even be envisaged as an adumbration of the field theory, once the so-called presentations are externalized. He even speaks of the "free space" granted to one idea at one time, to another idea afterward. Let anyone read, for example, Letter 14 of this series, and Herbart's achievement will be seen in a modern light.

HERMANN LOTZE (1817-1881)

In Hermann Lotze, Herbart had a successor at the University of Tübingen who was in some respects superior to him. Herbart's great contribution was largely in pedagogy, while Lotze was preoccupied with the basic connections between metaphysics and psychology; and in the latter, he dealt with the borderline territory between normal and abnormal psychology, which necessitated some exploration of the physiological foundations of the mental processes. As a doctor of medicine, he had gained an insight into the working of the nervous system which a philosophical training could not have afforded him. Johannes Müller and Helmholtz had already begun paving the way for the scientific revolution; and Lotze had drunk deep of the well of knowledge in several different fields. One of the scarcely known facts about his unexpected excursions is his spontaneous sponsorship of a society for the study of Yiddish literature, which in his day, was *terra incognita,* even to the Jews themselves.

Each of Lotze's works, the *Physiologie der Seele* (*Physiology of the Soul*), the *Medizinische Psychologie,* and the *Mikrokosmus,* was massive and contained solid material, scientifically anchored, despite his idealistic conclusions, which were beginning at this time to sound unprofessional for a laboratory man.

Lotze is known even to elementary students because of his doctrine of local signs, which purports to explain how we can refer certain sensations to a particular location in the body, but Lotze's service to psychology is far broader, even though it is not as universally accepted.

In the first place, he examined anew the problems of body and mind, and became the chief proponent of interactionism, influencing a number of psychologists even in our own time, the most important being William McDougall. His very detailed account of what goes on during an emotional state was perhaps the most satisfactory up to the time of Sherrington and Cannon. He was not afraid to defend views, such as the substantiality of the soul and the existence of faculties, which were beginning to drop out of psychological discussions.

Despite a hankering for metaphysics, Lotze may be regarded as one of the founders of modern psychology. There was still something of the mystic in him, but his scientific training and acute mind, ever alert to the discoveries of the day, saved him from overemphasizing the purely cogitative.

JOHANNES MULLER (1801-1858)—
Founder of Modern Physiology

While he was not a psychologist but a physiologist—the first in Germany to hold a chair in physiology independently of anatomy—Müller's influence on psychology was considerable. He was in his early thirties when his *Handbook of Human Physiology* appeared (1833), and it at once became a classic. It was here that we find the formulation of the doctrine of specific nerve energies, according to which it is not the particular stimulus but the special nerve and its termination in the cerebrum which causes the specific sensation.

Müller made many discoveries which impinged upon psychology. He recognized, for instance, that the psychophysiological process was sensory-motor. A series of experiments revealed the reflex nature in the spinal cord; and the arc-like action was seen to occur also in the higher cerebral processes.

In 1835, Müller, through a series of ingenious experiments with an artificial larynx, was able to prove that the vocal cords behaved in the same way as vibrating strings, and that the pitch differences were due to differences in tension of the cord.

Of equal importance was Müller's work on visual space perception. The problem was: Why do we see but a single object although each eye receives an impression. The stereoscope, which Wheatstone devised about this time, facilitated the steps to an explanation of the phenomenon.

Notwithstanding his pre-eminence in physiology, he adhered to the doctrine of a vital principle which shapes each individual's development, thus harking back to Artistotle's *entelechy*.

Müller's observations in various departments of psychology, even the affective life, were empirically handled and contained the germs of later experimentation, on a larger scale and under more technically controlled conditions. In the fifty-seven years of his life time, physiology became a full-fledged science, and with it, psychology began to move up in the scientific bracket.

FRANZ ANTON MESMER (1733-1815)—
Explorer or Charlatan?

Older readers can still remember when hypnotism was referred to as mesmerism. The later term "hypnotism" stems from the English physician, Braid, who was a pioneer in that field. Nevertheless, the fountainhead was Mesmer, an Austrian physician, who, as a showman, traveled extensively over Europe and elicited an interest among the educated in the various doctrines which he set forth. These theories were all vague, but since he was able to attract attention through his cures of hysterics through suggestions given the patient while in a hypnotic trance induced by passes, the practice and the underlying theory were for a time attached to his name.

The idea was not unknown in the Orient, but in Europe it was novel, so when Mesmer reached Paris, where big things were in preparation—for instance, the French Revolution—there was much ado in medical circles, and he took the city by storm. During the clinics or *séances*, hysterical women fainted, and the whole procedure had something awesome about it. A commission was appointed, one of its members being Benjamin Franklin, and the verdict was that no animal magnetism was involved, as Mesmer proclaimed, but that it was all a matter of physiological process.

Mesmer had been influenced by Paracelsus, who believed that the celestial bodies affected the weal and woe of mortals. He also appears to have received some information along those lines from a book by an English physician, Richard Mead (1673-1754), *De Imperio Solis ac Lunae* to judge from an examination of certain passages in that and Mesmer's *De Planetarum Influxu* (1766). At first the mesmeric force was associated with astrology, then it became identified with electricity, until Mesmer settled for "magnetism," which was differentiated from the physical sort by the qualification "animal," i.e., vital. The force was supposed to be cosmic and operated through certain individuals; and Mesmer rated himself high, if not highest, in that fortunate group.

Mesmer has gone down in the annals as a charlatan, but it is quite possible that he was an earnest practitioner, impressed by the mysteries of his experiences. While it is true that he operated with metallic gadgets, it is not certain that his motive was to deceive. In any case, he left a host of followers, and is one of the colorful figures in the history of the mental sciences.

His activities in Paris added to the gaiety of intellectual circles. A play, *The Doctors*, satirizing Mesmer and his adjutant, Deslon, had audiences, just prior to the Revolution, in stitches. The *baquet*, a sort of bathtub with mirrors and bars, around which the sitters would gather in a mediumistic formation, was the special target of the playwrights. Pinel, the foremost alienist of his day, attended a number of the meetings, even submitting to "magnetism," but he thought of the whole business as a farce; at most, a social event for the ladies and a bit of fun for the men who were holding their hands.

That hypnotism would play an important part in La Salpêtrière and Nancy, that it would be the basis of faith healing, that it would enable P. P. Quimby to cure Mrs. Mary Baker Eddy of her functional paralysis and thus inaugurate a new creed—all that was not dreamed of by either Pinel or Mesmer himself. What is more, in the last decade, hypnotism has come to be regarded as a respectable branch of medical psychology, serving as a means of diagnosis, as a convenient and practical anesthetic agency, and as a form of therapy in the milder neuroses. A regular journal in the United States, devoted to the applications of hypnotism in conjunction with other methods, has been publishing many interesting experimental and clinical papers.

"Hypnoanalysis" is the term used for a procedure combining hypnotism and psychoanalysis. In passing, it may be mentioned that Freud, as a graduate student in Paris, was very much interested in hypnotism, and as a young man, translated Bernheim's book on suggestion into German, but later abandoned the method entirely.

FRANZ JOSEF GALL (1758-1828)
Phrenology Takes the Field

Gall shares with Mesmer not only one given name but also a few of his less pleasant vicissitudes; and even the reputation which he left as a scientist shares the stigma attached to Mesmer. Less spectacular than his older contemporary, but certainly better endowed as an investigator, Gall, after making an extensive study of the brain, came to the conclusion that its various regions could be correlated with special functions of the mind. The convolutions were thus invested with a particular significance. Had he occupied himself with function in the sense of activity alone, he might have come upon the principle of brain localization, but his interest lay in complex mental capacities, such as memory, rhythm, love, and number; and thus he launched a new vessel which was to founder in the ocean of science—phrenology.

In accordance with this doctrine, the concentration of fiber clusters was supposed to show a high development of some special faculty, and even the outer conformation of the skull became a measuring area suitable for such diagnosis. The chart shows the topography of the brain in relation to the talents, propensities, and character traits which Gall rather arbitrarily drew up.

When he started giving his phrenological lectures in Vienna, controversy raged between him and his opponents; and soon enough, his foes were victorious, for the Austrian government prohibited the course as dangerous to religion. Gall benefited by the ban, since it aroused greater interest in his ideas, but in 1807 he decided to try his luck in Paris, and together with his disciple, Spurzheim, he began a series of physiological researches which redound to his credit as an investigator. These were published in a definitive six-volume edition between the years 1810 and 1819.

His science has been discredited by scientists in general, yet a few noted physicians took up the cudgels on his behalf even as late as the past generation, attempting to prove through portraits that composers had a special bulge around the ear, while mathematicians showed a protuberance elsewhere on the skull. Paul Möbius in Germany was inclined to subscribe to the doctrine, in modified form, while in England, the physician, Bernard Hollander, was its most ardent advocate. In the United States, Fowler became its chief propagandist.

ERNST HEINRICH WEBER (1795-1878)—
Founder of Psychophysics

Ernst Heinrich Weber, like several other physiologists, affected markedly the fortunes of psychology. He was working at the University of Leipzig on the muscle sense, which he was going to establish by means of experiments, when in the process of adding or subtracting a certain amount from a container which the subject held without looking at it, he stumbled upon the "just noticeable difference" that the subject was able to detect as *felt* rather than seen. This led to the formulation of Weber's Law, and later to Fechner's expansion of the law to take in the various senses, and to the establishment of a new branch in psychology, namely, psychophysics.

Weber was also instrumental in suggesting the local-sign theory which Lotze later formulated. This came about through a series of experiments Weber had conducted on double touch with compass points. On different parts of the body the double touch was felt as single, if not too close to one another, but on the tip of the finger, even a millimeter's distance was sufficient to distinguish the two points. The results of these experiments on the skin form demonstrative material in almost every elementary psychology class.

GUSTAV THEODOR FECHNER (1801-1887)—
Father of Scientific Psychology

Gustav Theodor Fechner may be considered the father of experimental psychology, although he would have been most surprised to learn of the honor. If Fechner had not given us his *Elemente der Psychophysik,* in 1860, psychology might still have become a science, but it was the impact of that work which brought to many the consciousness that here was at least a basis for a new science. Weber had prepared the material, but it was Fechner who worked out the implications and formulated "Weber's Law," as he dubbed it rather magnanimously. It ushered in a new era by spanning the bridge between the mental and the physical.

Psychology had been at a disadvantage in that it could not demonstrate laws. All mental states were fleeting. Only physiological conditions could be studied objectively. Fechner set himself the task of establishing a unit of measurement for the mind, and with the help of Weber's conclusions, amplified by his own extensive experiments, he found that there were ratios of sensation to stimulus, that these ratios differed in the various sensory spheres, and that the just noticeable difference in heaviness, brightness, loudness, or pitch could be taken as a unit of measurement, like the milligram or ounce in weight measurements.

It can well be understood that the new relationship found between the physical stimulus and the experienced sensation set workers in this field agog; and when Wundt founded the first psychological laboratory in 1879, most of the experiments turned around psychophysics. Not that Fechner's results were accepted universally—there were critics who were skeptical of the laws established, and, in fact, Fechner himself was not altogether sure whether the results were sufficiently uniform and consistent even in the separate senses to warrant the reference to a law. However, the ground had been broken for a new approach to psychology, and the methods which Fechner had laid down were applied and theoretically discussed for a whole generation. Fechner's formula, $S = K \log R$, in which S relates to the sensation and R to the stimulus, became the storm center for many a psychologist and physiologist. The assumption that a stimulus can be measured in a direct way, while the sensation is measurable only through the stimulus, was assailed as a piece of self-deception. When we speak of mental measurement at present we are generally alluding to tests of various types, but up to Fechner the very phrase would have been considered nonsensical, although Herbart was, indeed, puttering with formulae. It was Fechner who broke the ground and paved the way for the large projects which subsequently occupied the attention of experimentalists: physicists, physiologists, and psychologists alike.

It would be a gross mistake to suppose that Fechner's contribution began and ended in what he called "outer psychophysics." In a volume which he designated "inner psychophysics," he took up problems of after-images, memory, attention, sleep, and other topics.

If Fechner made a dent in the development of psychology as a science, he may be considered as the founder of experimental aesthetics through his *Vorschule der Aesthetik* (*Propaedeutics of Aesthetics*) (1876). He was seventy-five then, and had been an invalid nearly half his life, but rarely do we find a scientist or scholar who has produced so prodigiously in different areas of human endeavor. He worked steadfastly as a translator of a dozen French scientific manuals in order to supplement his pittance as a university lecturer. He brought out article after article in physics, physiology, and psychology; and, to boot, he wrote satires poking fun at the foibles of the day under the pen name of Dr. Mises. In 1821, when he was but twenty, he began the series by a so-called "proof that the moon consisted of iodine." No doubt in our day he would have made capital of vitamins and royal jelly and of course sputniks. At the age of thirty-eight, he suffered a nervous breakdown, which lasted at least three years, after which he resumed his labors with indefatigable avidity; and despite his physical complaints, he managed to live to a ripe old age. He will probably rank as the most significant psychologist known to us, on a par with Wilhelm Wundt.

Fechner was a romantic even during the heyday of his career, but as he turned from science to philosophy, which is the way of all scientist flesh, he indulged in speculations more in keeping with thinkers of the East. He spoke of the souls of plants, and believed that the world was animated. Indeed, his whole scientific period was interspersed with mystic sprees, during which he published a small book on life after death, *Zend-Avesta,* wherein he attempts to prove that souls are the property of all objects, and later *Nanna,* which, ironically enough, unlike Zola's novel of lust, was a discussion of plant souls.

It may be surmised that Fechner was a psychophysical parallelist of the monistic type, i.e., for him body and mind were identical, and only seen as separate from two different viewpoints.

HERMANN VON HELMHOLTZ (1821-1894)

Like his great teacher, Johannes Müller, Helmholtz was primarily a physiologist, but his contributions to psychology were immense. It would not be an exaggeration to rank him as the foremost scientist of his generation. Even physics was enriched as a result of his accurate methods and ingenious experiments; and while he began as a professor of anatomy and physiology at the University of Königsberg, he ended up as professor of physics at the University of Berlin.

There is something about his countenance which reminds us of Bismarck, but if they both had an iron will, the "blood" portion of the famous epithet could be said, in the case of Helmholtz, to have been replaced by "mind."

Students in their elementary course in psychology learn that, in 1850, Helmholtz was able to measure the rate of propagation of the impulse in the motor nerve of the frog, which had been considered too brief to be measured. In 1855, he discovered that there were summation tones, in addition to other combination tones. In 1858, on the basis of extensive experiments he advanced the theory that consonance is the result of a smoothly flowing sequence of tones while dissonance was due to beats between tones or overtones. In 1860, he formulated the theory of tonal qualities in vowels, regarding consonants as unanalyzed noise. His *Tonlehre,* which appeared in 1862, was a landmark not only in physiology but in psychology, for it is in this work that he developed the theory that it is the basilar membrane in the inner ear, consisting of a series of fibers of varied lengths, that responds to various notes. This resonance theory of hearing, "old stuff" now, was a revelation a century ago. He even traced the passage of sound waves up to the auditory nerve.

Helmholtz's work on optics was even more fundamental. In 1862, he invented the ophthalmoscope in order to study the retina and its refractive properties directly. He then found the mechanism of accommodation through the elastic contraction of the lens. His *Handbuch der physiologischen Optik* is a voluminous work which is a mine of firsthand information on everything relating to the eye and vision. Here we have the elaboration of the Young theory of color vision as due to three separate organs in the eye, giving rise to red, green, and violet, and other colors when stimulated in combination.

Helmholtz's ideas on space perception, the function of double images, the role of unconscious inference in the interpretation of visual cues, and his improvement on the Wheatstone stereoscope, are further evidence of the man's gigantic achievements. No one has so enriched our knowledge of the so-called higher senses and their workings as Hermann von Helmholtz.

EWALD HERING (1834-1918)

Ewald Hering may be considered, in a sense, the counterpart, if not the rival of, Helmholtz, even if he did not attain the same stature. Like Helmholtz, he was a physiologist, known to the elementary student in psychology because of his theory of color vision, which differed from Helmholtz's in positing four instead of three primary colors, operating in either a building-up process (green, blue) or a tearing-down process (red, yellow). Nearly all the phenomena of color vision (complementary colors, after-images, white, black) are explained on this basis.

Although both theories offer difficulties, Hering's seems to be the more satisfactory of the two, and in the most recent experiments on vision, Hering's name is beginning to figure more prominently than in past decades, when he was overshadowed by the greatness of Helmholtz.

Hering's application of anabolism and catabolism to the other senses, for example, to account for the sensations of warm and cold, was less fortunate, since it was later discovered that there were different skin spots for the two sensations.

Hering did not see eye to eye with Helmholtz in the matter of space perception. The latter was an outright empiricist, and set out to build up space perception from various cues we receive, while Hering was what was later known as a nativist. Apparently, he held with Kant that the notion of space is of native origin, and that total perception cannot be derived from particulars which are not like it. One can understand why Hering is regarded as one of the pioneers of Gestalt psychology. He was always dealing in totalities and relationships, rather than in sequential and piecemeal steps. The latter method appeals more to the young student because of the ingenuity involved in the explanation. It is only in more recent times that the global aspect has appeared in a new light.

Hering's nativistic leaning is probably the reason for his radical view of memory; for as early as 1870, he made a stir with his address before the Vienna Academy, "On Memory as a Function of Organized Matter." He attributes memory to paper, which if creased will tear better; or to wood, which if punctured will better take a nail. Even William James appeared to be intrigued by this objectivistic doctrine, which may be the foundation of modern learning theories, particularly those behavioristically interpreted.

"A MAN NAMED WUNDT"

Writing to Thomas Ward in 1867 from Berlin, where he was visiting courses, William James, then a young man of twenty-six, had the following to say about the science which he was to establish twenty-three years later on a solid footing:

> It seems to me that perhaps the time has come for Psychology to begin to be a science—some measurements have already been made in the region lying between the physical changes in the nerves and the appearance of consciousness. . . . I am going to study what is already known, and perhaps may be able to do some work at it. Helmholtz and a man named Wundt at Heidelberg are working at it and I hope, if I live through this winter, to go to them in the summer.

Wilhelm Wundt's name will be associated not only with *the founding of the first psychological laboratory in* 1879, at the University of Leipzig, but with the training of a large number of European and almost as many top American psychologists. Leipzig seemed to be the Mecca of all American students in this field, and Wundt for half a century was, if not the prophet, at least the high priest, of the new "faith."

Aside from the experimental impetus which he imparted to psychology, he may be rated as its greatest systematizer. He was, however, more than that. There is scarcely a topic, whether sensation, emotion, feeling, perception, or language, to which he did not contribute something of his own, and what he did not tackle, his outstanding students worked on.

Born in 1832, in the state of Baden, Germany, he managed to live beyond the end of the First World War, publishing during sixty-eight productive years, as E. G. Boring figured out in his *History of Experimental Psychology,* 53,735 pages. We may be quite certain that no psychologist has broken this record. When we consider that his works were largely technical and required a tremendous amount of research, we can appreciate the extent of his prolificacy.

After receiving his M.D. degree, he turned to physiology and was fortunate in becoming the assistant of the great Helmholtz at Heidelberg. His physiological period resulted in a textbook. Then came a manual of medical physics. At the same time he was occupied with more psychological problems on an experimental basis. When he went to Switzerland as incumbent of a chair in inductive philosophy, after failing to receive an expected promotion in Heidelberg, he had already completed his *Physiologische Psychologie* (1873-74) which, in its six editions, was to serve as the standard work for advanced students through two generations.

Almost as elaborate were his works on logic, ethics, and philosophy as a system. Perhaps his most ambitious work was the *Völkerpsychologie* (*Collective Psychology*), which took nearly twenty years to complete, and if Wundt had done nothing else but turn out these ten bulky volumes, he would have his niche in the forefront of psychology. In this truly *magnum opus* he deals with myth, religion, language, and art as the expression of the folk, and it is almost awesome to contemplate the mountains of facts which

Wundt was able to assimilate and systematize in advanced age. One of his characteristics was the extraordinary patience with which he kept constantly revising his work. There is hardly a doctoral dissertation, even in the American universities, which he did not exploit in making his revisions.

Wundt's personality was not on a par with his mental endowments. Although his students, who later gained distinction on their own merits, such as Kraepelin, Lipps, Titchener, J. M. Cattell, Pace, and Scripture, evinced an admiration for him, he was capable of antagonizing associates through personal animus.

William James disliked him, though as a young man he had looked forward to working with him; and a lifelong opponent of Wundt's was Carl Stumpf, of the University of Berlin. Both James and Stumpf were inclined toward nativism and global points of view, in common with the later Gestalt psychologists, while Wundt, like his teacher, Helmholtz, was an empiricist, building up a total situation out of individual cues. This approach appeals to the physical scientists, but not to those who see the interstices as well as the bricks, and are unwilling to lose sight of the whole while analyzing it.

It was partly because of Wundt's rejection of perhaps his most brilliant student, Hugo Münsterberg —who dared to refute the master's conclusion that we are aware of our muscular innervations—that the twenty-nine-year-old psychologist received a call to Harvard by William James, in 1892. Wundt's most devoted disciple, E. B. Titchener, was later invited to found a laboratory at Cornell. The two laboratories were at loggerheads with one another, although Titchener and Münsterberg did not differ fundamentally in theory. Both were orthodox in their views of mind, the former a thoroughgoing structuralist, the latter veering toward functionalism, being interested in use and action. As a system builder, Wundt was naturally a structuralist.

It is quite likely that Wundt will go down in history as the central figure in psychology, because of both his contributions and his influence as a teacher of subsequent psychological leaders.

CARL STUMPF (1848-1936)—Foremost Nativist

Just as Helmholtz had a lesser rival in Hering, so Wundt had his counterpart in Stumpf, who did not make the dent in psychology that Wundt did, but who, because of his position as professor at the University of Berlin and his persistent experimental work, must receive a prominent place in even a brief survey of psychology.

Born in a village in Bavaria, in 1848, a decade after Wundt, he received an excellent musical education, in addition to the usual collegiate studies, and might have ended up as a composer or instrumentalist but for the family tradition.

At the University of Würzburg, he came under the influence of Franz Brentano, a remarkable personality, whose medieval detachment and courageous stand brought him many admirers, although his *Psychology from the Empirical Standpoint* (1874), a modernization of the Aristotelian-Thomistic act-and-faculty psychology, was for a long time his only major work.

Stumpf's interest was in the fundamentals of both philosophy and psychology rather than in building up a system of psychology, as Wundt almost succeeded in doing. Wundt was a psychologist who also cultivated the field of philosophy, while Stumpf was a philosopher who did important spadework in psychology, devoting nearly a lifetime to the exploration of such phenomena as tones and melody.

His theories, based on countless experiments, were

nativistic. Unlike Helmholtz and Wundt, he did not believe that our perceptions were built up piecemeal out of elementary fragments interpreted in terms of past experiences, which is the genetic or empiristic point of view. He resembled William James who, in common with him, stood for global representation. (The reader of James will remember how he denied that the taste of lemonade is compounded of the taste of lemon and the taste of sugar, etc.) Stumpf went even farther than James when he rejected the latter's theory of emotions, which is more in keeping with a compounded view, akin to the genetic.

Stumpf gave a slightly different turn to Brentano's *act*-psychology, and called it *psychic* function, which to him is the true substance of psychology, though there are other "ologies" which must be taken up at a tangent, since they intervene. Such things as colors, images, and tones constitute the study of phenomenology, while a study of the relations between psychic contents falls under the heading of "logology," and a more obscure division is called "eidology."

To what extent these hair-splitting classifications were of value, except as mental training, cannot be established, and while at present no psychologist makes use of them except in historical context, the fact that *Gestalt psychology* originated in Stumpf's laboratory in Berlin, where Wertheimer, Koffka, Köhler, Lewin, and Hornbostel brought out some remarkable facts about perception, points up the importance of Stumpf's teachings. Thus, in a sense, Carl Stumpf may be said to have been the godfather of Gestalt psychology, as well as the chief experimentalist on tones.

EBBINGHAUS (1850-1909)—Pioneer in Memory

Every beginner in psychology has heard the name Ebbinghaus, even if he seldom spells it correctly in examination blue books.

Born in a small place near Bonn, in 1850, his education was the usual one in Germany, with philology as a major. He then shifted to philosophy. He served in the Franco-Prussian war, resumed his studies at the University of Berlin, and then traveled on the Continent, studying and teaching intermittently, until he discovered in a Paris *Bouquinerie* a copy of Fechner's *Elemente der Psychophysik,* which brought him something like an illumination.

Prior to Ebbinghaus, much had been written on memory, but experiments were at best few and far between. Here was his chance. Without the opportunities which others had had in the environment of the founding psychologists, he set to work to apply, in a general way, Fechner's method to the measurement of memory. In order to rule out meaning so as to keep conditions uniform—the minimum requirement of experimentation—he devised the system of nonsense syllables (two consonants with a vowel in the middle) and for years he used them upon himself as subject, bringing out his classic *Ueber das Gedächtnis* (*On Memory*), in 1885.

Most of the results were significant. We know that learning must be distributed rather than crowded, that the more repetitions, the better results, that overlearning can result in a prolonged memory, that associations may be formed or reinforced with back material as well as with the material following; and

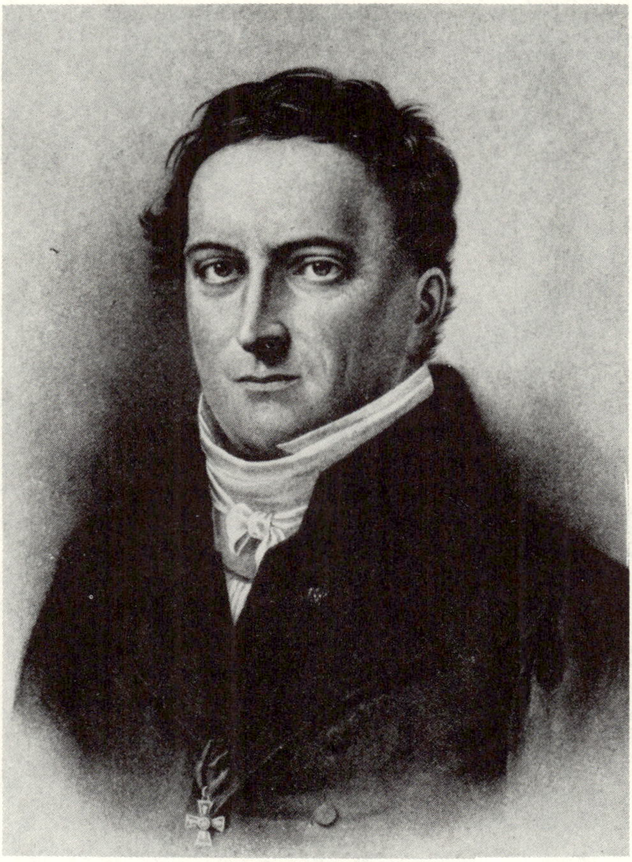

Johann Friedrich Herbart

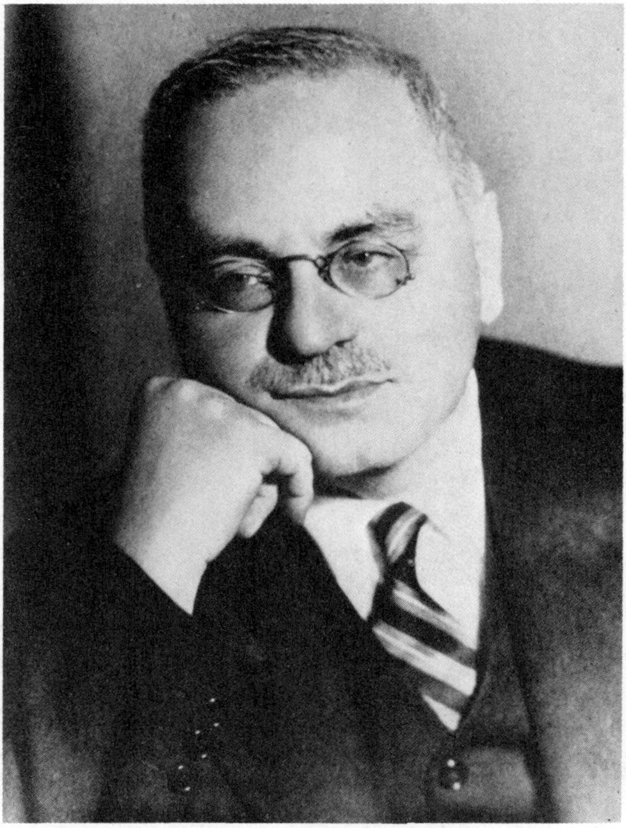

Alfred Adler

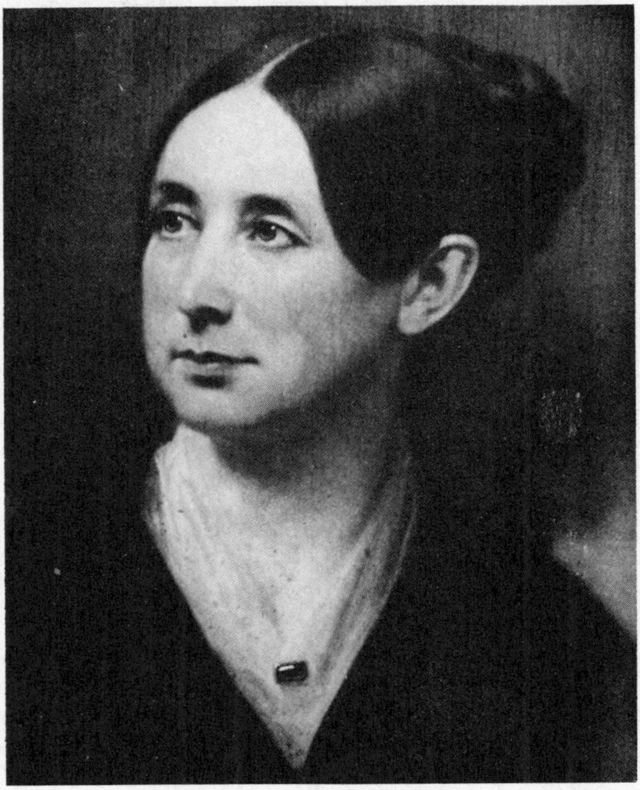

Courtesy New Jersey State Hospital

Dorothea Lynde Dix

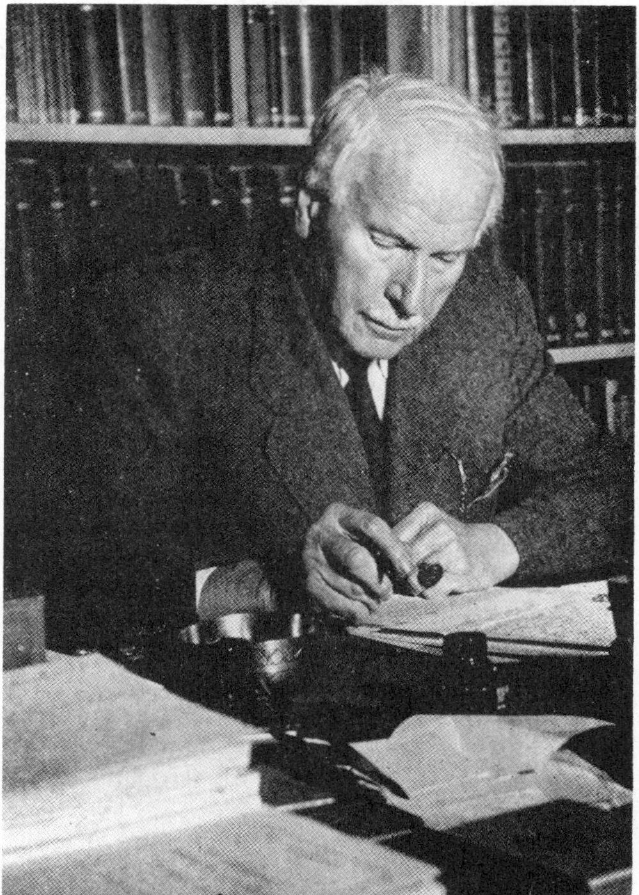

ATP-Bilderdienst

Carl Gustav Jung

that the association is not only between close syllables, but the more remote syllables in a given series become linked too. He even plotted, tentatively, a forgetting curve. Had Ebbinghaus not undertaken the nerve-racking task, we might have had to wait for some other patient investigator. Ebbinghaus was not content to reach conclusions from merely one extended series of experiments. He had to repeat a number of them to satisfy his scientific conscience.

In 1890, he co-founded one of the most important journals combining psychology and sensory physiology, with an impressive editorial board, outshining the earlier Leipzig journal founded by Wundt.

Ebbinghaus is known in psychology also as a pioneer in mental testing; for in 1897, he published his results with the analogy test, or as it was later called the "completion test"—one of the most effective indicators of intelligence. A sample is: "July is to May as Saturday is to——— [Thursday]." * In personality, Ebbinghaus, although not so versatile and ingenious, reminds one of Binet, and like him, his life was short. He died at the age of fifty-nine, while revising his first volume of a textbook which in point of lucidity and literary flavor was of a piece with William James's *Principles of Psychology*. A radiant personality, prepossessing in appearance and co-operative, he was practically the antithesis of Wundt.

G. E. MULLER (1850-1934)
Simon-pure Experimentalist

While Johannes Müller, the great physiologist, occupies an honored place in the psychological textbook, his namesake, G. E. Müller, is scarcely mentioned, and yet, according to E. G. Boring (*History of Experimental Psychology*), "As a power and an institution,

* Actually Ebbinghaus did introduce a completion test, where words omitted in a given passage had to be filled in from the context.

he is second only to Wundt." This estimate may be slightly exaggerated, inasmuch as Boring is apt to be partial to a man who was wholly engrossed in experimental work at a time when his colleagues indulged in much theorizing, and were even devotees of philosophy.

Born in 1850, and receiving the usual loaded humanistic education, his erudition began to pall on him before he was twenty-one. Going from Leipzig to Göttingen, where he came under the influence of the illustrious Lotze, whom he succeeded a decade later, he threw himself into experimental psychology with a vengeance, and with Schumann and Pilzecker, took up the work in memory from where Ebbinghaus left off, and presented the psychological world with significant results. He and his students found more effective ways to learn (whole piece plus specific items), discovered the associative and retroactive inhibitions, devised new methods such as that of paired associates in learning, rigged up more reliable apparatus, made use of a lightning calculator who had a phenomenal memory, and in addition, furthered our knowledge of color vision, space perception, and attention.

In short, even if Müller's claim as a *proxime accessit* to Wundt on the experimental level may remain unproved, his three volumes of monographs have meant much more for the development of psychology than twice that many textbooks. At least a dozen of his students became leading psychologists, and thus his influence was deeper than might appear at first blush. One reason for his unpopularity was his temperamental outbursts in controversies. Men who evolved systems were not to his taste. He turned out excellent parts, and was capable of making the most of his advantages. Under him, the Göttingen laboratory became as much of an experimental center as Leipzig or Berlin, attracting among others D. Katz, E. Rubin, and O. Kroh.

OSWALD KULPE CREATES THE WURZBURG SCHOOL

Würzburg could never rate as a first-class institution, according to German standards, but it was Oswald Külpe (1862-1915) who put it on the scientific map.

While his predecessors and contemporaries were busying themselves with the sensory processes, he, mentally more akin to Stumpf in that he was drawn to philosophy and aesthetics, directed his attention to the psychology of the higher mental processes, or what we generally call thought.

Under his guidance, a number of able investigators probed what goes on while we are thinking. Such terms as "determining tendencies," "conscious attitudes," "mental set," "uniformity of psychic act," "imageless thought," hardly convey to the layman what intensive experimentation was necessary to bring to the surface such potentials.

Naturally, because the sphere of operation (thought) lent itself less to objective observation than, say, sensation, memory, or perception, the Würzburg conclusions were often questioned, but in the heyday of introspective psychology, they could not but make a profound impression in scientific circles. Among his best-known students were such noted psychologists as Ach, Messer, Marbe, Watt, Orth, and Karl Bühler. Only Bühler, who settled in the United States after the advent of the Nazis, survives.

L. WILLIAM STERN (1871-1938)—The Personalist

Starting with a contribution on folk psychology, Stern afterward switched to experimental psychology, wrote and edited some important monographs on the psychology of testimony, and then by systematizing the known data on individual differences, established the branch of differential psychology. His original work on child psychology and intelligence tests (the phrase "intelligence ratio" i.e., "quotient" is of his coinage) has put him in the front rank as an investigator of educational psychology, and two of his books in this field have been translated into English.

He later dropped the concept, maintaining that there is no monosymptomatic diagnosis of personality, but that the person must be approached from various angles, of which intelligence testing is only one.

Next to Münsterberg, he stands out as the pioneer in applied psychology, particularly in Germany.

He founded the *Zeitschrift für angewandte Psychologie* (*Journal of Applied Psychology*), as well as its monograph series, organized the Hamburg Institute for Applied Psychology, and was one of the editors of the *Zeitschrift für pädagogische Psychologie.* Although he was the chief authority on applied psychology in Germany, he also earned a world-wide reputation as a philosopher through his three-volume *Person und Sache* (*Person and Thing*). As professor of psychology at Hamburg University he trained a number of students who later showed his influence in their work.

Stern belongs at the antipodes of behaviorism. On the surface he resembles Titchener, but the latter was an arch-elementarist, building up the higher complexes of mind out of sensations, images, feelings, and perceptions, while Stern begins with a highly complex and seemingly abstract concept of the person. To him the person is a totality which can be studied through the experiences according to a given scheme.

Stern believes that the person is goal-directed and in that respect he is an ally of McDougall, but he also stresses the person's creative phase. For this reason he cannot agree with the Gestaltists, who deal with perception rather than with the perceiver.

Stern was president of the German Psychological Society and was conducting a meeting, when Hitler's appointee arrived and ordered him to vacate the chair. His dismissal came in "due" course, and he soon migrated to the United States, where McDougall found a place for him on the faculty at Duke University. His textbook appeared in English translation, but its success was equivocal.

Both McDougall and Stern died within months of each other at the same age.

KARL BUHLER (originally, Bühler)

Perhaps the last of a generation of pioneers is Karl Buhler, who, though German-born (Baden, 1879) and trained (M.D. at Freiburg and Ph.D. at the University of Strassburg), is chiefly spoken of as an Austrian psychologist since from 1922 to 1938 (when he was dismissed by the Nazis because of his Jewish wife, Charlotte, a leading child psychologist) he headed the Department of Psychology at the University of Vienna.

Thereafter he taught in Norway, and in 1939 migrated to the United States, where he had been visiting professor twice before. Presently he has been working as a consulting psychologist at the Cedars of Lebanon Hospital in Los Angeles.

Buhler is primarily a functionalist. As an assistant of Külpe at Würzburg, he experimented on the thought processes. In the early revolt against associationist theories, he worked on the Gestalt principle, and defended the thesis that humans and animals develop and perceive configurations.

His systematization of the phenomena of language and expression has been of great value to the psychologist. Similarly, his textbook on child psychology, antedating Piaget's standard books, emphasized his biological orientation and has had a number of revisions.

Animal psychology, particularly the communication system, has also been a fruitful field of research for the versatile Buhler.

Buhler has been opposed to all mechanistic theories, such as behaviorism, as well as to psychoanalysis. His concept of "function pleasure," which is derived from play and creative work, is not to be identified with the "satiation pleasure" which is a principle of Freud's system.

The Gestaltists

Out of the Berlin and Göttingen laboratories arose a new school in psychology, the seed of which was planted by C. von Ehrenfels (1859-1932) in Prague, who was puzzled over the recognition of two series of notes, played in two different keys, *as the same melody*. Evidently the notes or the elements were not all that mattered. The totality was not, as William James observed, simply a summation of the components, but something over and above.

In Göttingen, G. E. Müller had already developed a *Complex-theorie,* which dealt with similar problems, and under his direction, Edgar Rubin and David Katz carried out some fundamental experiments, but it was Max Wertheimer (1886-1943) who first came to grips with the paradoxes of movement and perception in general, beginning the work at the University of Berlin, where Kurt Koffka, Wolfgang Köhler, and E. V. Hornbostel were working on investigations along the same line. Later, Kurt Lewin joined them, and when the group subsequently founded a journal (*Psychologische Forschung*), Kurt Goldstein, the neurologist,[4] joined them, and since they were nearly all Jews, the Brown Plague drove them to escape to the United States. Even the non-Jew, Köhler, found it expedient to leave the great university in Berlin, where he succeeded Stumpf, and join the faculty of a small, although high-rating American college (Swarthmore).

Max Wertheimer was not prolific, never made it

a point to produce *en gros,* but worked whenever the spirit moved him; and then it would be play to him. Thus the toy stroboscope and the tachistoscope yielded some important results in connection with our observation of movement.

Through a series of ingenious experiments with lines and dots, figures and background, the Gestaltists were able to establish the triumph of the whole over the parts, the fact that in actuality our minds are prone to unify and read into isolated marks, if not too far apart, a definite relationship. We tend to close small gaps in circles or quadrilaterals (*closure* phenomenon), and we read into random marks specific meaning, as if they were objects or definite symbols.

Wertheimer was not only an able experimentalist, but strong on epistemology, with a grip on logic and mathematics. Köhler's forte was the area of physics, and while interned, he carried out a number of experiments on apes, which argued for the possession of insight on the part of some infrahuman species. Köhler delved into the fundamentals of systematic psychology and attempted to show the place of value in the Gestalt theater.

Koffka (1886-1941) may be considered as the chief exponent of the system, especially in the genetic field. Child development and learning are interpreted in terms of totality and consciousness as against the fragmentation and sheer behavior mechanisms of the stimulus-response psychologists. Gestaltism opposed itself mainly to every form of behaviorism, including the later stage denominated operationism, while psychoanalysis was practically ignored. The libido, so vivid and colorful and ubiquitous in the Freudian camp, figures so punily in the domain of the Gestaltists that it attracts no attention. For them the unconscious holds neither fascination nor terror. It is a different child we see through Freud's colored glasses and through Koffka's and Lewin's frosted spectacles—or perhaps binoculars, since Lewin's field theory, dynamic though it is, cuts across spatial rather than temporal areas; and the brand designation "topology" which Lewin borrowed from mathematics indicates to what extent "place" is stressed in his system.

Kurt Lewin (1890-1947) was the methodologist of the group, a resourceful experimenter with a minimum of apparatus. Concentrating on the sphere of personality and motivation, he extended his methods from child psychology to what he called group dynamics, applying the same principles to serve his ends. His diagrams were especially helpful to elucidate his hypotheses.

Kurt Goldstein (1879-), a neurologist of considerable experience, exploited the biological field and treated the organism as a whole—all the psychophysiological functions depending upon, and not merely constituting, the nature of the totality.

While Edgar Rubin, late Director of the Psychological Laboratory at the University of Copenhagen, was one of the early experimenters to bring out the significance of the configuration (Gestalt) he stood somewhat apart from the movement. His fellow student and close friend, David Katz (1884-1953) who became Director of the Laboratory at Stockholm, continued to make important contributions in various departments and gave a clear and comprehensive account of the school.

In consequence of the Nazi restrictions, all the Gestalt leaders settled in the United States, and it is here that the movement began to thrive. The *Gestaltian* protest was instrumental in plowing up the soil anew and proved an antidote to the unfounded assumptions transmitted from one generation of psychologists to another. That Gestalt psychology is not in the limelight at present is only natural. Much of it has been absorbed in the textbooks, and thus it is taken for granted.

ETHNIC BRANCHES
B

BRITISH PSYCHOLOGISTS

In a book in which only the highlights can be considered, emphasis must be upon men who were in some way pioneers. Locke, Berkeley, Hume, and Brown were discussed earlier because, in their time, all psychologists were primarily philosophers, and they made basic contributions to psychology. They were pathfinders.

The same consideration cannot be accorded the Mills (James and John Stuart), though they consolidated the facts on associationism, and were responsible for a theory which was later dubbed "mental chemistry," according to which experiences are atomized and synthesized, the acme of empirical psychology.

CHARLES DARWIN (1809-1882)
Trail-blazer of Evolution

If one wonders why Darwin, a naturalist and geologist, is found among the psychologists, it should be remembered that Darwin wrote a classic on the *Expressions of the Emotions in Man and Animals.* Aside from that, however, his impact on the mental sciences has been tremendous.

Darwin actually was not the originator of the doctrine of evolution, but he was its greatest exponent. The principle itself was propounded by his contemporary, Alfred Russel Wallace, and was hinted at even in antiquity. Darwin's greatness stems from his establishing the theory, and meeting all criticism, in fact anticipating a good deal of it, and leaving no stone unturned until he was satisfied in his own mind that he had proved his point.

Phrases like "the survival of the fittest," "natural selection" and "struggle for existence" are as significant in the sphere of psychology as in biology, and affected all fields of thought.

It is in the area of genetic and comparative psychology that Darwin's work occupies a special place of honor, even if his views are not altogether acceptable. His leaning toward Lamarckianism has not found favor in the eyes of scientists, who are convinced that acquired characteristics are not transmittable. Nor did his continuity argument, which would raise the level of animal intelligence, thanks to an anthropomorphic interpretation of, say, a dog's or baboon's behavior, sit well with more critical experimenters like Lloyd Morgan. However, Darwin's conception of *adaptive function* played an important role in understanding the evolution of typical behavior and the organs which were responsible for it, such as the dilation of the nostrils and curling of the lips and baring of the teeth in rage. When it was urged that such adaptiveness could not be detected everywhere in emotional expression, Darwin retorted that sometimes the expression was a hangover from a time when it was necessary. An emotion with a biological basis may have an opposite with no biological significance. The response is simply the opposite of the other. For example, self-assertion is biologically grounded; self-abasement is not similarly useful, but the law of opposites brings about a response which is the opposite of that of self-assertion by a sort of organic association.

Whether or not we can justify Darwin's stand in full, there is no question that it aided the introduction of the functional aspect in psychology. People began to look for a purpose, for utility, in both organs and behavior. Thus Darwin contributed greatly to the subsequent development of psychology.

Herbert Spencer's two-volume textbook *Principles of Psychology,* first published in 1855, was excellent in applying the theory of evolution to the explanation of physiological and mental processes, but as a psychologist Spencer went no farther than Brown of the Scottish school. Similarly, Bain was a philosopher who did a good deal of psychologizing. Sully made good surveys of psychological theories. James Ward, also a philosopher, who became well known through his lengthy article (afterward extended into a book) in the ninth edition of the *Encyclopaedia Britannica,* was perhaps, the first in England to take a stand on orientation in psychology, and engaged psychologists in other lands in controversy. Ward might have been a good critic, but he accomplished little that was to be lasting. George Stout could write useful and literary compendia like his *Analytic Psychology,* in two volumes, or his *Manual of Psychology,* without adding much substance to the discipline, except as a critic.

The real work came from men like Charles Darwin (*Expression of the Emotions in Man and Animals*), G. Romanes, and C. Lloyd Morgan, whom we shall consider in the section on Animal Psychology.

The Many-Sided FRANCIS GALTON (1822-1911)

It is not until we reach Francis Galton that we find one of those universal minds out of which almost anything can sprout. Like most of the British intellectual giants, he taught nowhere, and was not bound by tradition, profession, or the need to earn a living, having been fortunate in his ancestry, and in his relatives, for Darwin was a cousin of his. J. McK. Cattell speaks of him as "the greatest man I have known."

Galton was an independent man in every way. He had a powerful build, enjoyed good health, and remained active physically and mentally almost to his ninetieth year.

A roving researcher, Galton would occupy himself with various problems, not necessarily psychological, as the spirit moved him, and whatever he undertook seeemed to yield something of value. He was the first to report on types of imagery (*Inquiry into Human Faculty*). He invented the Galton whistle, which is used in connection with the discrimination of overtones, and in order to establish extremes of pitch. He investigated the relationship of fingerprints and character. He wrote on color blindness, on memory span, on composite portraits, and on many other topics—in each case not contenting himself with armchair observations, but conducting actual experiments, not on a large scale, it is true, but sufficient to open up a new area. His investigation into genius, and his finding that heredity is its chief explanation, impelled him to create a new movement—eugenics.

Galton was the true polyhistor, and whether he tackled anthropology, psychology, or geography, he was bound to come up with something which could not be brushed aside as trivial.

His interest in genius and eugenics led him to make a serious study of statistics, which he was obliged to apply to biological data, and thus he became the pioneer in biometrics, which he bequeathed to a disciple better suited to grapple with the mass of data, namely, Karl Pearson.

WILLIAM McDOUGALL (1871-1938)

In the opinion of the writer, William McDougall was not only the foremost British psychologist but the man who made the greatest contribution to the science in all the English-speaking countries. One naturally thinks of William James as the great pioneer of scientific psychology in the United States, but it can scarcely be denied that McDougall tackled many more problems independently.

William McDougall may be regarded as a scion of the Scottish School, although he was reared in the English tradition of Bain, Ward, Stout, and Shand. Cambridge, Oxford, a year at Göttingen, and a four-year internship at St. Thomas Hospital gave him an unusual background.

Two generations of students came under his tutelage at the University of London, and at Oxford, Harvard and Duke Universities, and at the time of his death a score of books, of unequal merit, attested to his productivity in almost every branch of psychology.

His *Primer of Physiological Psychology* was a model of condensation and exposition. He is known chiefly for his *Introduction to Social Psychology*, which passed through some twenty-five editions and impressions, and in which his theory of instincts, linked with the emotions, received formulation. He boldly espoused the doctrine of a soul in his *Body and Mind*, as a result of which he began losing caste among the experimentally minded. When his sponsorship of psychical research became known, his stock, despite his appointment to William James's chair at Harvard, began to drop; and all his subsequent books, including the *Outline of Psychology* and the *Outline of Abnormal Psychology,* could not restore his erstwhile prestige. The parapsychological activities at Duke University have no doubt been inspired by him.

McDougall's psychology is called *hormic,* the central idea being that there is an end or purpose which goads us to action, without any real knowledge of its nature, and often without benefit or even thought of pleasure. A general striving, therefore, and not cognition, or even feeling, is at the root of all animal activity. The mechanisms or dynamisms through which the purpose is achieved or sought are the instincts. Human progress can be explained only in terms of the "horme" or "drive."

The mind is not a series of momentary events, but possesses a permanent organization, which acts upon the physical just as the bodily processes affect the mental (*the doctrine of interactionism*).

McDougall's chief difficulties lay in proving, or even explaining, interactionism in a physical world; his belief in free will; and his commitment to the theory of the transmission of acquired characteristics, which he sought to demonstrate by experimenting with generations of rats, a procedure which most experimentalists did not take seriously.

Whatever his shortcomings, McDougall was a good experimentalist, a better systematizer, and a brilliant theorist. As a dynamic psychologist, he ranks next to Freud, whose genius he appreciated without accepting his tenets. Since his death, there has been a growing tendency to rehabilitate him, to the point of reviving his doctrine of instincts, which was so repugnant to American psychologists in general.

CHARLES SPEARMAN (1863-1945)—
and Factorial Analysis

Though his name is not as well known as McDougall's, Spearman brought up a whole school of pupils who used and elaborated upon his statistical methods, which came under the general heading of factorial analysis.

It must not, however, be thought that he was a statistician rather than a psychologist. His first love was philosophy, but before he could do much with it, a military mission diverted him. "As for these almost wasted years, I have since mourned as bitterly as ever Tiberius did for his lost legions."[5] Though he carried an assortment of philosophical and psychological books from one military station to another, he did not begin to live intellectually until he struck Leipzig where that titan, Wundt, was supreme.

After receiving his doctorate, he went to Würzburg, where Külpe attracted many promising students, and after three months there, he turned to Göttingen and the very different G. E. Müller.

In 1907, he received an instructorship (or, as they called it there, a "readership") in experimental psychology at the University of London, where he remained until his retirement, gradually developing the factorial analysis school, and training a corps of young statisticians and educational psychologists.

Spearman's chief work was concerned with the nature of intelligence. According to him, intelligence is an energy which manifests itself in a general phase

(G) and through specific outlets (s). The specific factors were left to a number of graduate students to discover. The doctrine of two factors in the operation of intelligence was accepted by most psychologists in England and by many elsewhere, but it has also had some very powerful opponents, such as Titchener at Cornell, the whole Gestalt school, Thorndike at Columbia, who fashioned a multimodal theory, and, of course, the behaviorists, who rejected all references to mind, restricting psychology to reactions to stimuli.

To Spearman, intelligence consists of the *eduction* of relations, and in this he may be regarded as a functionalist who validates his findings through mathematical formulae. His work on the correlation coefficient (rank formula) and what has been called the "Spearman-Brown prophecy formula" has become fundamental in all educational measurement. Here we can see his kinship with Galton, who influenced Spearman in the same degree as did Wundt.

Spearman did not produce many books. His works include *The Nature of Intelligence* and *Principles of Cognition* (1923), *The Abilities of Man* (1927), and *Psychology Down the Ages,* in two volumes (1937), which is a history not of psychology but of selected problems that lead up to the general discussion of ability and temperament, culminating in the two-factor theory, with the *pros* and *cons* threshed out in his favor. As he sees the situation, "at one extreme, statistical zealots have accumulated masses of figures that remain psychologically senseless. At the other extreme no less ardent typologists have been evolving an abundance of psychological ideas with little or no genuine evidence as to their truth." (Vol. II, p. 281). The outlook, however, is brightening, thanks to better understanding between both camps.

Spearman's students who, through correlations, have been discovering a number of specific factors like fluidity (f), perseveration (p), verbal aptitude (v), stamina (w), oscillation (o) and mathematics (m) have been applying their findings to education, psychiatry, and other fields. Spearman, who began as Grote Professor of Philosophy at the University of London, was succeeded by his most outstanding student, Cyril Burt, as Professor of Psychology.

W. H. R. RIVERS (1864-1922)

W. H. R. Rivers, who had studied medicine and was drawn to physiological research, having, together with Henry Head, come to the conclusion that there were two types of cutaneous sensations—protopathic and epicritic, the former more primitive and vague than the latter—later developed into a field anthropologist, working with William McDougall and C. S. Myers among the Torres Straits Islanders.

He later turned to the study of dreams and the unconscious, and became interested in psychoanalysis. His three best-known books are *Dreams and Primitive Culture,* (which may be regarded as a bridge leading to Geza Róheim's more comprehensive investigations), *Instinct and the Unconscious,* and *Conflict and Dream,* which was published after his death.

Rivers was not a famous psychologist, but he exercised considerable influence on his students. Sir Frederic Bartlett, who came under his influence, writes, in a private communication, that Rivers would continually warn him about getting immersed in affairs. "It was advice which he signally failed to apply to himself."

Just as Rivers was plunging himself into productive work, after giving up the editorship of the *British Journal of Psychology,* he died before a surgeon could be found on a holiday to operate on him, in his college rooms at Cambridge.

CHARLES S. MYERS (1873-1946)

Charles S. Myers, not to be confused with F. W. H. Myers (1843-1901), perhaps the leading spirit in the psychic research movement in England (whose *Human Personality and its Survival of Bodily Death* [1903] can still be read with profit), was associated with both Rivers and McDougall in the Torres Straits expedition, and later engaged in experimental work, first at the University of London, and then at Cambridge University, where he brought up a generation of empirical psychologists and brought out, in two volumes, the most serviceable laboratory manual in English. As editor of the *British Journal of Psychology* for over a decade (part of the time jointly with Rivers), he strengthened the experimental phase of psychology in England, which had been neglected up to that time.

Myers was an able organizer. It was he who arranged for the first International Congress in Psychology, held at Oxford in 1923, and was its first president. He soon turned his attention to industrial psychology, and was largely instrumental in the founding of the National Institute of Industrial Psychology, with a formidable roster of titled sponsors. In his autobiographical sketch, Myers has the following to say of his organizing and administrative work: "My interests and talents in the latter direction are related probably to my ancestors' business careers . . . but in thus following my early inclinations and natural bent,

I have probably served psychology better than I could have done in other, more usual, ways."

Myers was not a theorist. It was primarily as a methodical worker and director of research in the practical sphere that he takes his place in the history of British psychology.

Taking his cue from Rivers, of whom he speaks in terms of admiration, he set store by the results gained from an examination of individual differences rather than the dwelling on mass data.

As may be surmised, Myers was not concerned with mind-body problems. Activity was his domain; and so he can be rated as a functionalist, with measurement of activity as his goal. In the field of applied psychology in Britain, Myers occupied a position similar to that of Hugo Münsterberg, although nowise to be compared with him in other respects.

FREDERIC CHARLES BARTLETT (1886-)

Frederic C. Bartlett, unassuming as he is, devotes only a dozen pages in his *History of Psychology in Autobiography* to his own life and activities. He accomplished more than is evident from this skimpy sketch, which deals principally with his views on psychology, and how these took shape.

Always generous in his appreciation of others, he speaks of the impact of Stout's textbooks, Ward's book-size article in the *Britannica,* and the teaching of Rivers and Myers, to whom he refers almost with reverence. It was through Myers' efforts that a psychological laboratory worthy of the name was built at Cambridge University, and Myers was an experimentalist teacher of no mean order.

Even if Bartlett had done little else than complete the investigation on remembering, he would have earned his laurels as a leading psychologist.

In this work, he has gained interesting results through a series of ingenious experiments, his forte consisting in a superior methodology and sound interpretation, based not on a foregone conclusion couched in an imposing hypothesis, but on an analysis of the factors involved. As a critical observer who deals with the situation as a whole, Bartlett has few equals among contemporary psychologists. It was not quantity bolstered by statistical formulas so much as diversity of variables which intrigued him, to the extent of examining the mnemonic achievements of aborigines in a primitive setting in Africa. Furthermore, he was the first to treat of memory in a social light.

The fact that his first publication was entitled *Exercises in Logic* and his latest *Thinking: an Experimental and Social Study* should give us a clue as to his orientation. Logic and society are the rails on which he has been traveling.

His other books include *Psychology and Primitive Culture* (the impetus toward anthropology coming from Rivers and Myers), *Psychology and the Soldier,* as well as a number of studies in symposia and commemorative volumes. Bartlett had a large part in the revision and enlargement of Myers' experimental textbook.

For about a quarter-century he edited the *British Journal of Psychology,* writing, in addition, hundreds of reviews, which were both concise and judicious, models of crisp evaluation.

During both world wars Barlett significantly assisted the cause of defense, and was knighted in 1948, being the first experimental psychologist to be thus honored. He was also the first to be given the professorial title in psychology at Cambridge. In 1932, he was elected a Fellow of the Royal Society, and has since won numerous citations and honorary degrees.

CYRIL BURT (1883-   )

The foremost authority in Great Britain on tests and juvenile problems, Cyril Burt was knighted for his work in the field of education, in 1946.

A doctor of science, with a good chemistry and philosophical background, acquired at Oxford, he taught at the University of Liverpool and the University of London, until his retirement in 1950, and was engaged in many administrative offices, particularly during the Nazi war.

An expert on statistics, he was one of the editors of the *British Journal of Psychology*, and brought out books on *Mental and Scholastic Tests*, *The Young Delinquent*, *The Subnormal Mind*, *The Backward Child*, among others, and wrote extensively for periodicals.

His views are hereditarian in the main, with a psychoanalytic side-glance. In his major work, *Factors of the Mind* (1940), he has this to say of the purpose of his school.

> In my view, the primary object of factorial methods is neither causal interpretation nor statistical prediction, but exact and systematic description. And I suspect that most of the confusion has arisen because factors, like the correlation coefficients on which they are based, have been invoked to fulfill these three very purposes and so here made their appearance at three very different levels of thought. (p. 13)

C

FRENCH PSYCHOLOGISTS

If France has not contributed half so much to the science of psychology as Germany, it is perhaps because the affections played such a prominent part in French tradition, beginning with Descartes.

Thus, France had her pioneers in abnormal psychology, but her psychologists were interested primarily in cases rather than in generalizations and laws. French psychology, unlike its German counterpart, was not grounded in physiology, nor allied with physics and chemistry, although it did have points of contacts with medicine, such as it was at the time. Charcot, as we shall see in another connection, was a psychiatrist. Charles Richet (1850-1935) did graduate from physiology, and his productivity was immense on a variety of subjects, but his influence on the course of psychology, even in France, was negligible. That of Ribot, on the other hand, was considerable.

THEODULE RIBOT (1835-1916)

Perhaps the first in France to concentrate on psychology proper was Théodule Ribot who, ninety years ago, brought out a survey of contemporary British psychology, followed, about a decade later, by a similar study of German psychology. Though his book on psychological heredity shows him in the light of a genetics investigator, Ribot appears mainly in the role of historian and expositor, and as such acquits himself creditably, a fact soon proved by the demand for German and English translations.

Ribot also has the distinction of being the first to teach a course in experimental psychology in a French University (Sorbonne). Before that, however, he devoted several years to the publication of his studies on abnormality in memory, volition, and personality, which are the best known of his works. Thus, he too followed the French tradition in its concern with disorders, though Ribot dealt with them more systematically than anyone of his predecessors.

Ribot's subsequent works attest to his growing interest in the experimental and biological phases of psychology. An important work for that period was his *Psychologie de l'Attention;* and his *Psychologie des Sentiments* was followed up by *La Logique des Sentiments, Essai sur les Passions,* and *Problèmes de Psychologie Affective,* all of them pointing to his characteristically French preoccupation with the feelings and emotions. That feelings had a logic of their own was something of a novel idea, and, in a sense, foreshadowed one of the tenets of psychoanalysis. His books on the evolution of general ideas and his essay on creative imagination combined a good deal of stimulating thought based on numerous instances culled from biography and personal experience.

His last work, *La Vie Inconsciente et les Mouvements* (1914), bore evidence of his switching from a sensory to a motor emphasis, which began with Stricker in Austria, and James and Münsterberg in the United States. Ribot's approach evidently continued to dominate French psychology, since Janet found behavior, or as he called it "conduct," to offer the most adequately descriptive psychological category. To Ribot's credit must be reckoned the founding of the *Revue Philosophique,* which accommodated psychologists as well as philosophers.

ALFRED BINET (1857-1911)—
Genius of French Psychology

The most important name in French psychology is without doubt that of Alfred Binet, who trained for law, but never practiced it. Charcot's magic wand at La Salpêtrière attacted him like many others, but his was too universal a mind to be wholly preoccupied with abnormal psychology. His tribute to that field was paid in his book on alterations of personality (*Les Altérations de la Personnalité*), which came out in 1894, but as early as 1885, he had already busied himself with problems of the higher thought processes that even Wundt's laboratory did not take up. *La Psychologie du Raisonnement* appeared in 1886. Next came his pilot work on the psychic life of micro-organisms, followed by his *Introduction à la Psychologie Expérimentale.* In 1900, appeared his book on suggestibility.

As chief of the Psychological Laboratory at the Sorbonne, he was constantly conducting experiments, whether in chess playing, lightning calculation, psychography, or individual differences; and everywhere he made shrewd observations to guide future research. He also founded the first psychological journal in France, *L'Année Psychologique.*

It was, however, his work on defective children and the intelligence tests associated with his name which brought him everlasting fame; for through these, the educational world acquired an instrument for measuring intelligence. Even if credit is also due his collaborator, Théodore Simon, the architect of the whole scheme was Binet, who kept improving and revising the scale after its first appearance in 1905.

PIERRE JANET (1859-1947)

Janet is best remembered as the founder of the dissociation school in psychopathology, but his long and productive life, which began with instruction in philosophy, took on various phases, and in his last decades we find him turning out volume after volume in general psychology.

Coming under the influence of Charcot, at about the same time that Freud studied with the French master, he soon discarded the accouterments of hypnotism, as did Freud, and forged a theory of his own, explaining neurasthenia and psychasthenia in terms of the depletion of energy. Janet claimed that Freud merely changed the nomenclature, but that is incorrect. An entirely different point of view, rooted in libidinal ties, dominates Freud's system.

Janet's specialty was observation and description rather than interpretation. His sympathy is with objective psychology, and while he cannot be called a behaviorist, he approaches the physicalistic camp. His books on hysteria and psychotherapy have augmented his reputation but have not made any disciples for him.

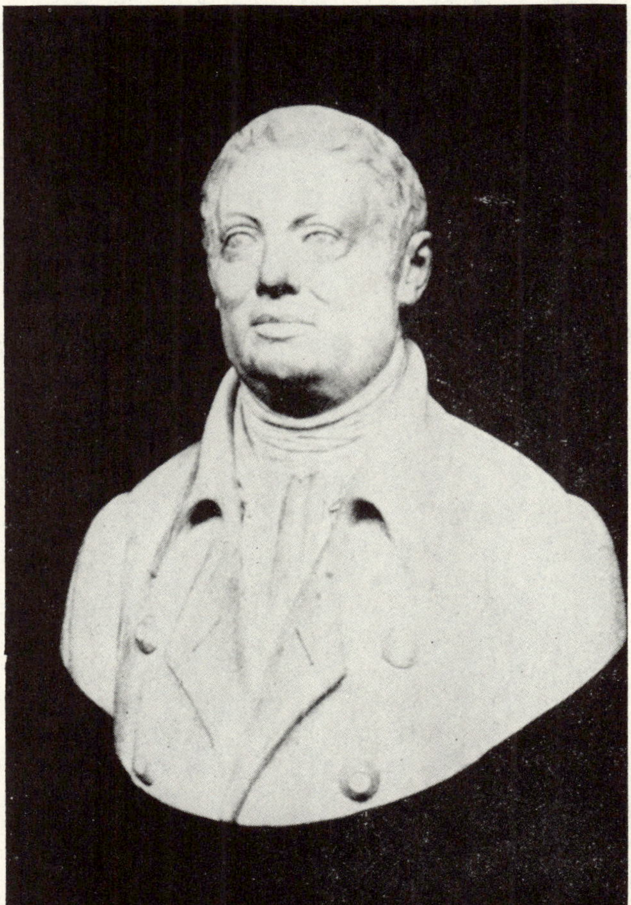

Vincenzo Chiarugi

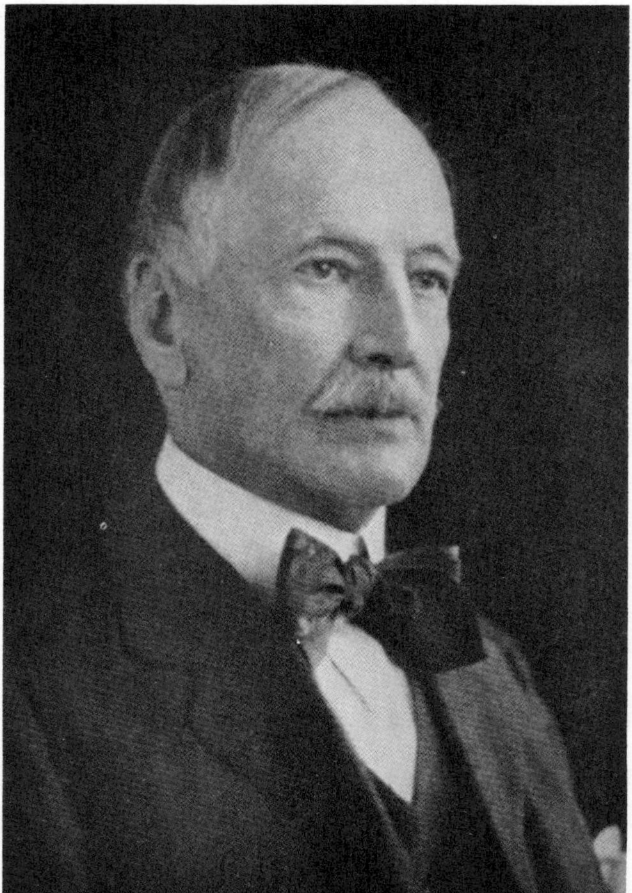

Morton Prince

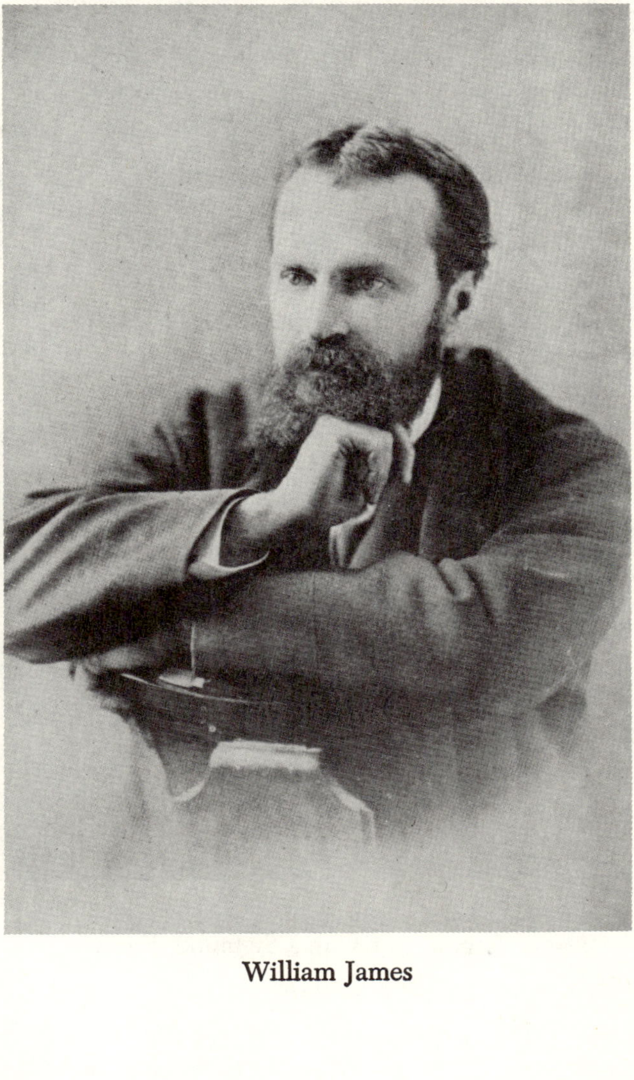

William James

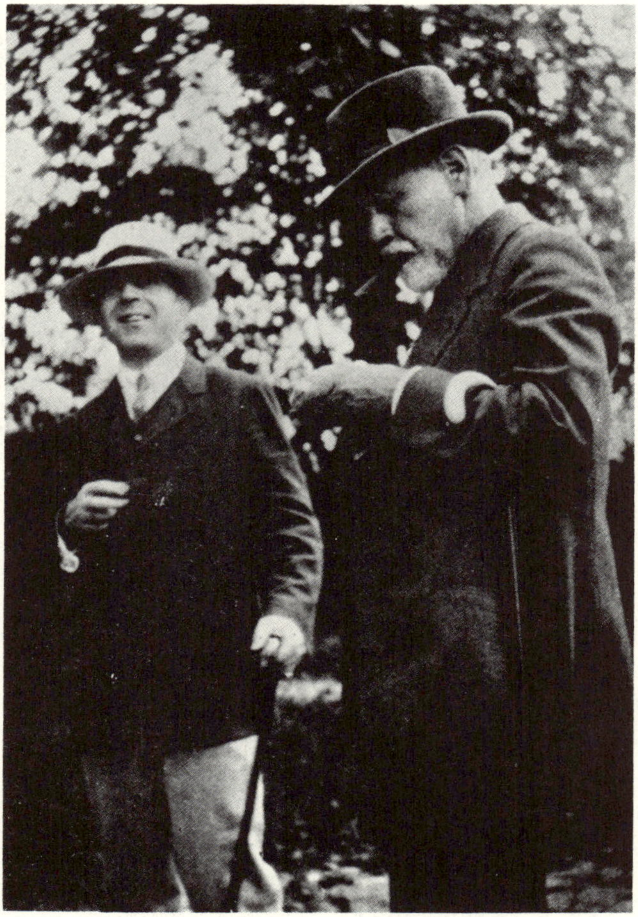

Courtesy Ernst Freud

Ernest Jones and Sigmund Freud

H. PIERON (1881-   )

Since the realm of the abnormal and peripheral matters (social phenomena) loomed so large in French psychology, the experimental side was generally neglected. Not that there were wanting experimentalists, but their level of aspiration was much lower than that of the German experimentalists. They were not so long-nerved, and their interests were diffuse.

In Henri Piéron, we have an experimentalist who is both broad and thorough. He might be regarded as Binet's successor or epigone. In the first place, his grounding in physiological psychology rendered him partial to carrying on research in sensation. His chief work is *Le cerveau et la Pensée,* which was translated into English. His *L'Evolution de la Mémoire* (1910), *Le problème physiologique du Sommeil* (1912), and *Psychologie expérimentale* bring to bear an objectivistic slant on subjects which, in France, had been handled rather speculatively. Piéron might be regarded as an operationist of sorts.

As the chief experimentalist in France, it was fitting that he should have been the incumbent of Binet's office as Director of the Sorbonne Psychological Laboratory. He also succeeded Binet as editor of *L'Année Psychologique.*

There are, of course, other Frenchmen who gravitated to psychology from other fields and who made important contributions: Durkheim, the ace sociologist; LeBon, the group psychologist, whom we shall meet later; Lévy-Bruhl, the philosopher (primitive mentality); Charles Richet, the physiologist, who could say that nothing human was foreign to him; Georges Dumas, who burrowed in side paths, but whose voluminous *Traité de Psychologie* brought together the specialized contributions of a number of psychologists and provided France for the first time with her own handbook—no mean accomplishment, though not to be compared with the stupendous *Traité International de la Psychopathologie* which A. Marie edited and brought out in 1912-14.

GEORGES DUMAS (1866-1946)

Georges Dumas did not influence French psychology in the manner of Binet, Ribot or Janet, but he contributed greatly to it. His training was not only in medicine but in the humanities as well.

Born in 1866, in Ledignan, he acquired doctorates in letters and medicine, and in 1912 was appointed professor at the Sorbonne. Together with Janet, he founded the *Journal de Psychologie*. In consequence of his experience as a psychotherapist during the war, he published an important work on mental and nervous disorders due to the war (1919). His work on sadness and joy (*La Tristesse et la Joie*), 1900, constituted his doctor's dissertation for the doctorate in letters, and he had already brought out books on Tolstoi and the philosophy of love (1893), the intellectual states of mind in melancholy (1894), and *The Smile*, psychologically and physiologically considered. Probably his chief service to French psychology consisted of editing two massive volumes of the *Traité de Psychologie* (1923, 1924), which he had taken eight years to put into shape and which thus far has been superseded in France only by that of Marie.

A capable organizer, Dumas made it his business to promote French public relations in other countries, chiefly in South America (Argentina, Chile and Brazil).

He may be said to belong to the school of Ribot, but as a physician he stressed the neurological and psychopathological aspects of the psyche. His Latin thesis on what Comte felt about the psychology of his time revealed his critical spirit (he later took up the two positivist "Messiahs," St. Simon and Auguste Comte in a separate volume—1906). His point of view is best characterized as approaching the clinical one of present-day psychology.

D

ITALIAN PSYCHOLOGISTS

Psychology has never made much headway in Italy. There have been distinguished criminologists, alienists, or psychiatrists, physiologists like C. Lombroso, G. Sergi, who made inroads into psychology; but only G. C. Ferrari, Sante de Sanctis, A. Gemelli, F. Kiesow, and perhaps Vittorio Benussi may be cited as having become known outside Italy. Of these, De Sanctis and Gemelli have been the most outstanding.

It is noteworthy, too, that no one university had the edge on the other in this respect. There was no tradition handed down, no school, except in the case of Lombroso, who was primarily a neurologist and founder of criminal anthropology.

G. C. FERRARI

G. C. Ferrari at the University of Bologna did much for the mentally ill and juvenile delinquents in Italy. He apparently was a good organizer and could make useful contacts. It was he who translated James's great textbook and it was he who founded the first Italian psychological journal, the *Rivista di Psicologia.* His laboratory was a modest affair—altogether different from Gemelli's in Genoa—nor did he have the catholic interests of De Sanctis; but there is no denying that he exerted a beneficial influence on the advancement of the mental sciences in his country. The only jarring note in his autobiographical sketch is the fulsome praise which he showers upon Mussolini, whose "war diary" he published in his *Rivista,* in 1915-16.

SANTE DE SANCTIS (1862-1935)

Sante De Sanctis studied medicine, and for some time practiced as a physician. Rome in the early nineties was a true scientific center, with men like Sergi and L. Ferri stimulating research. Young De Sanctis studied with Forel at Zürich, and in Paris he profited by his association with men eminent in medical psychology, so that he was a well-rounded scientist when he began teaching in the university. He soon began to acquaint himself with the work of Freud, whom he did not follow in all implications, although he admired his genius and accepted many of the Freudian mechanisms.

De Sanctis was a researcher and extremely productive. His chief interest was, naturally, in psychopathology: dementia praecox, the neuroses, hysteria. The feeble-minded next captured his attention, and he produced a series of studies dealing with all kinds of defectives. He wrote on attention (his principle of "paraprosexia" is really the principle that excessive consciousness of an impulse will tend to inhibit it). He wrote on dreams and on expression peculiar to thought. He did not believe in the bodily causes of mental disorders. A series of experimental investigations were published under the head of *Psicologia Sperimentale,* which, as might be anticipated considering the culture, stressed criminology. Experimental psychology was applied in the Rome laboratory; for De Sanctis remembered Cuboni's maxim,

"Hold fast in the scientific field but seek liberty beyond."

De Sanctis' autobiography is a perceptive and objective self-analysis, with a number of striking reflections.

MARIO PONZO (1882-1960)

De Sanctis was fortunate in his successor at the University of Rome, Mario Ponzo, who was born in Milan, received his medical degree at the University of Turin, and eventually became Director of the Institute of Experimental Psychology at Rome.

His main work, consisting of hundreds of papers, was in the field of sensation: taste, smell, the thermal and cutaneous senses, but he had spread himself over many different areas. Illusions, testing, and more particularly applied psychology, occupied his attention in later years. For some time he had been regarded as the chief representative of Italian psychology.

AGOSTINO GEMELLI (1872-1959)

The most energetic of the Italian psychologists, whose laboratory most resembled the American laboratory in the variety of investigations which were open to graduate students, was curiously enough a Franciscan monk who had turned from militant socialism and materialism to devout Catholicism and Scholastic thought, even founding the Rivista di Filosofia Neo-Scolastica.

Like Ferrari, Kiesow, and De Sanctis, he had a thorough training in physiology, working under the Nobel Prize physiologist, Golgi, and in Germany under Verworn and Edinger; while Driesch and Hertwig were his teachers in biology, after he had earned his medical degree in 1902. After following up experiments along the lines of Sherrington and Pavlov, testing the validity of the James-Lange theory of emotions, he found himself gravitating to psychology and came under the tutelage of Kiesow, in the University of Turin, who, in turn, suggested that he study with Külpe at Bonn. He returned to teach at Turin, becoming professor in 1914, when as a result of World War I he took to testing military personnel.

At the close of the war, he founded together with Kiesow a new journal, devoted to psychology, neurology, and psychiatry, and in 1921 he founded the Università del Sacro Cuore at Milan. Practically destroyed by bombs during World War II, it was soon rebuilt and began to thrive as probably the most important psychological center in Italy, attracting students from many countries, the United States included. There is hardly a field which was not explored in Gemelli's laboratory, and the sixteen volumes of the *Contributi del Laboratorio di Psicologia* are a tribute to the dynamic priest whose Catholic orbit seems to have imposed no obstacles to the probing of phenomena in the spirit of, and through the methods of, modern science.

F. KIESOW (1858-1941)

It is questionable whether F. Kiesow should be called an Italian psychologist, though he taught at the University of Turin from 1899 until his death, first as an instructor in general physiology under Mosso, and then as a lecturer in experimental psychology, and from 1906 as professor of experimental psychology.

Kiesow's antecedents were German with, possibly, as his name would indicate, a Slavic infusion. His training was decidedly German, and having been among the early students of Wundt at the University of Leipzig, he was soon working on taste sensations, publishing his results as a doctoral dissertation.

Kiesow's interest in physiology brought him in contact with the eminent men of the day, von Frey, Ludwig, and Hering, and since von Frey had written a book on the pulse, and Mosso in Turin had succeeded in devising a method for recording pulse and breathing processes, Kiesow decided to go to Turin to familiarize himself with Mosso's technique and instruments. He came and saw and stayed, absorbed in the experiments with the ergograph, sphygomomanometer, and plethysmograph. The plethysmograph, we must bear in mind, was the basis of our lie-detector.

Kiesow's German training, not only under the physiologists mentioned, but under Külpe and Meumann as well, was fortunate for the development of Italian psychology. Although Kiesow admits to a mystic bent and even studied Hebrew sufficiently to read some of the Old Testament and indulged in fantasies about Jesus' activities in Jerusalem, he conducted his laboratory on a scientific level and counted many brilliant researchers among his students, the best-known of whom was Agostino Gemelli.

Kiesow was not as prolific as either De Sanctis or Gemelli, but he had a critical mind, and remained a follower of elementaristic (structural) psychology, as propounded by his first master, Wundt. To Külpe's views he was sympathetic; and he tested out the claims of the eidetic school on a thousand children, without finding the types distinct enough. Gestalt psychology, he thought, was too circumscribed to revolutionize the Wundtian system.

E

DUTCH PSYCHOLOGY
GERARDUS HEYMANS (1857-1930)

Although Gerardus Heymans was primarily a philosopher, who contributed to almost every branch of his discipline—theory of knowledge, ethics, metaphysics, aesthetics—there can be no doubt that he belongs to the outstanding psychologists in Holland.

It is a pity that he was not asked to write a sketch of his psychological activities for Volume I of the *History of Psychology in Autobiography.* The philosophical presentation which was included in Volume II was a translation from the German sketch prepared for a different purpose, and therefore devoid of psychological references, which ought to have been added editorially, since he died before the volume was in preparation.

For a key to Heymans as a psychologist, we have the answer to the opening question which he puts, namely, just what differentiates his researches from those of most of his contemporaries? His reply is that he employs empirical methods only to arrive at anti-empiristic conclusions. In that statement there is much truth. Methodologically, he is a rigid scientist, and yet he sponsors a general philosophy of psychic monism, which means that he represents the universe as consisting of consciousness, of which we partake as individuals. Thus his philosophy is based on a psychologistic postulate, because, according to him, it requires fewer assumptions than the epiphenomenalistic view, which borders on materialism, or the double aspect of mind and matter, such as Spinoza's psychophysical parallelism.

Aside from teaching at the University of Groningen, he conducted a number of investigations, on inhibition, individual differences, personality elements, the psychology of women, dreams, character, etc. His stress on primary-and-secondary-function types (Otto Gross) and independence of judgment are characteristic.

HENDRIK ZWAARDEMAKER (1857-1930)

In Hendrik Zwaardemaker, who was born and died in the same years as Heymans, we have a specialist whose name was known to almost every undergraduate because of his experiments on olfactory sensations, by means of the olfactometer which he invented.

Trained in the medical sciences and becoming an army surgeon, he was appointed, at the age of forty, to the chair in physiology at Utrecht left vacant by Engelmann, who had gone to the University of Berlin to replace the celebrated DuBois-Reymond.

Zwaardemaker, whose first study on odors was published in his twenty-first year, thought of mixing odors as we mix colors, and he succeeded in placing all odors into nine classes (afterward reduced by the German psychologist Henning to six). In these experiments, he used a large number of subjects of different age, sex, and status.

Zwaardemaker was not a mere experimentalist. He considered various hypotheses in relation to the senses, e.g., he thought that in animals the world of smell might be analogous to our world of the higher senses.

Nor did he confine himself to the sense of smell alone. In a soundproof room in the Utrecht Psychological Laboratory, he conducted a series of experiments in audition. He wrote a textbook in physiology, which went into several editions; occupied himself with problems of psychological energetics, suggested by new discoveries in physics (radioactivity and electronics); and was fascinated by Pavlov's studies of the conditioned reflex. But he thought "the comparative method finds its limit" in that the dimension of time is gradually becoming integrated with the other dimensions; and that another, that of the logical sense (concrete and abstract ideas), will in time be added.

E. D. WIERSMA (1858-1940)

A close collaborator of Heymans, Wiersma followed the pattern of the continental psychologists who were trained in the medical sciences. He was more the laboratory man, and his published papers range all the way from pure physiology to psychopathology, with a variety of intervening stations. A joint study with Heymans of the parts played by emotionality, activity, and secondary function in the development of neurosis is one of his most important ones, but he has also worked on heredity, mental tests, psychic inhibition, statistical methods, physique and race, sex differences, psychology of confusion, and the behavior of misers and spendthrifts.

GEZA REVESZ (1878-1955)

Curiously enough, it was a Hungarian Jew, Géza Révész, who was the leading psychologist in Holland; and the volume of his creative work, painstaking and brilliant as it was, entitles him to a central place in twentieth-century psychology.

The son of a vine-grower, in Hungary, he studied law at the University of Budapest, but on attaining the doctorate in jurisprudence, he went to Göttingen, where G. E. Müller directed the psychological laboratory, and then to the University of Berlin, where Stumpf and Du Bois-Reymond were his teachers.

Returning to Budapest, he became an instructor in 1908, but in 1914, he was mobilized as an officer and soon was in charge of military personnel matters. He had just been appointed full professor when General Horthy's regime made it impossible for him to carry on, and he practically fled to Holland, where Heymans in Groningen and Zwaardemaker in Utrecht gave him the research facilities he needed. But Révész required more of an arena.

He left for Amsterdam, where a municipal college was forming, and there he founded a laboratory of his own. In 1932, the University invested him with the first professorship in psychology; and in short order, Révész had a Psychological Institute, and in addition to the *Zeitschrift für Psychologie,* which he co-edited, and a Dutch psychological journal, which he had founded, he co-founded with David Katz, *Acta Psychologica,* an international journal of note.

Révész's interests and labors extended to the following fields: general psychology, vision, hearing, space perception, music, and especially genius and talent—which he was one of the first to investigate adequately—medical psychology, educational psychology, child psychology, animal psychology, language and thought, interpretation of the human hand (not palmistry), psychology of the blind, social psychology, and applied psychology. He wrote in several languages, and his versatility was extraordinary—he could even play Mozart from memory. Despite his versatility, Révész covered his subject thoroughly, and as an experimentalist showed ingenuity and sound judgment.

F

BELGIAN PSYCHOLOGY

While it is true that Belgium produced the father of modern anatomy (Vesalius) and psychiatrists of the order of Guislain, we should hardly expect a national trend of psychology to develop in a small country that is continually torn between two cultures, which she has been trying to synthesize in a mold of her own. Of the few universities in Belgium, that at Louvain, Catholic in spirit, was the one where psychology held a central position.

Actually, we might begin with the historical textbook (*Origins of Contemporary Psychology*) by Cardinal Mercier, who was, however, primarily interested in theology and philosophy. He reminds us of the theologian-psychologists of the early American era; for like them he was a remarkable administrator and just as liberal, as well as a great personality. It was he who founded the Institut de Philosophie at the old University, and as early as 1894, he procured Armand Thiery, a former student of Wundt at Leipzig, to organize a laboratory. It was there that Albert Michotte, the best-known Belgian psychologist, began to specialize in this field.

ALBERT MICHOTTE (1881—)

Albert Michotte was fortunate to study not only under Cardinal Mercier but also under van Gehuchten, a noted neurologist. He later rounded out his studies with Wundt at Leipzig and Külpe at Würzburg. It was the latter, along with Binet, who made a lasting impact upon his course in life. Wundt's cut-and-dried formulae and elementaristic postulates did not go well with Michotte's Catholic predisposition. For Michotte saw the necessity of scrutinizing an upper level of relations as well as the lower sensory units, and thus he appears to have come close to an *Act Psychology.* One of his early studies (together with E. Prüm) was on the immediate antecedents of voluntary choice. He was led to take up a dynamic position which made provision for unconscious processes.

After Louvain was burned down during the First World War, Michotte worked at the University of Utrecht, in Holland, in Zwaardemaker's laboratory. Subsequent experiments brought him closer to the results of the Gestalt School, but he was not ready to stop with the perception of form. To him, the *intrinsic meaning* was basic. At the same time, he became interested in the direction behaviorism was taking, and combining the aims of the two schools, began experimenting on motor processes from a Gestalt angle, supplementing the exclusively sensory preoccupation of the Gestaltists.

Michotte's long series of experiments displayed

great ingenuity in their setup as well as in methodology. They were concerned not with the minor problems of rhythm, memory, reaction time, and the like, but with such matters as "phenomenal permanence" or the differentiation between reality and unreality, or else testing out Hume's psychological interpretation of causality.

Michotte is a familiar figure at the international psychological congresses and has been the moving spirit of interlaboratory co-operation.

G

SWISS PSYCHOLOGY

THEODORE FLOURNOY (1854-1920)

Whether Théodore Flournoy was the scientist his pupil and successor, E. Claparède makes him out to be, in a whole monograph (*Archives de Psychologie*, Nos. 69-70, May-Oct., 1921), there is no denying that he was the pioneer in Swiss psychology.

Like many eminent men in Switzerland, he came from a family which had fled France because of religious persecution. To some extent he reminds us of William James, who was one of his close friends. In the beginning he, too, was not certain of his goal. At the University of Geneva, he entered the faculty of science, and received the bachelor's degree in the mathematical sciences. Despite the impact of men like Carl Vogt, he pondered spiritual problems and entered the University's divinity school, even taking up the difficult study of Hebrew; but soon spotting the drawbacks inherent in such a career, he switched to anatomy and physiology at Freiburg and Strasbourg, completing his doctoral thesis in 1878. But he did not practice; and in 1878, we find him a student of Wundt in Leipzig, where the first psychological laboratory was about to open. After a short stay in Paris, he returned to Geneva to embark on a long teaching career, which began in philosophy and ended in psychology—the reverse of James's experience.

In 1891, the chair of physiological and experimental psychology was created, and Flournoy insisted that it be affiliated with the faculty of science rather than with that of philosophy. His laboratory was founded in 1892, and investigation was begun on a number of problems (reaction time, sensation, ideation). But what primarily occupied his mind was psychic research, parapsychology; and his experiments with various mediums, principally Hélène Smith, made him at once the high priest of occult research, and almost the alter ego of the great American psychologist. His *From India to the Planet Mars,* translated from the French, into several languages was one of the sensations of the time. Newspapers in France, England, the United States, and other countries devoted pages to the "revelations" of Mlle. Smith, and in 1900 the famous Camille Flammarion was interviewed about the possibility of interplanetary travel. Flammarion, be it noted, was partial to the occult. At any rate, it is interesting to look into the expressions which the medium claimed to have gotten from her control, Leopold, and to examine Flournoy's rationalistic interpretations.

At about the same time (1901) together with Claparède, Flournoy founded the first Swiss psychological periodical, *Archives de Psychologie,* which is now edited by E. Piaget. His parapsychological preoccupation did not prevent Flournoy from presiding at the Psychological Congress held in Geneva, in 1906, an event which would be unthinkable at present.

EDOUARD CLAPAREDE (1873-1940)

Edouard Claparède (a native of Geneva, and of French Protestant descent) was a worthy successor of his cousin, T. Flournoy, who was in a sense his mentor, and with whom he later co-edited the *Archives de Psychologie.* In his autobiography, he makes a point of telling the world that although he could trace no German nor Anglo-Saxon ancestors in his lineage, he admired German thoroughness (*Gründlichkeit*). Another uncle, bearing the same name, had been a professor of comparative anatomy, whose lectures were praised by William James when the latter was a student in Geneva in 1859.

Claparède was destined for psychology. Early in life he made the acquaintance of Binet through an article on colored audition. Like other aspirants, he studied at Leipzig, and then took his medical degree, but instead of entering practice went to Paris, where Déjerine put him on the staff of La Salpêtrière. At staff conferences, there was more talk about the Dreyfus affair than about the patients, Déjerine, eminent psychiatrist though he was, antagonizing the students by saying that even if Dreyfus (then a wretched prisoner on Devil's Island) was innocent, and a true patriot, he would take the blame just to put a stop to the agitation which was so detrimental to France. Claparède significantly remarked that he could see how the logic of the feelings could betray both the reason and heart of a good man.

Still in his twenties, he had published a book on

association in which he took the biological stand that he never abandoned. His view on sleep was that it was the expression of a protective instinct, so that we would not become exhausted to the breaking point. This theory led to further elaboration in connection with hysteria and schizophrenia, in which he antedated the positions of Kraepelin and Kretschmer, although he received no mention in their books.

His wide interests included animal psychology (monograph on C. Bonnet and investigation of the Elberfeld horses), experimental pedagogy (his textbook was used in American colleges), and vocational or aptitude tests. A familiar figure at international congresses, he resembled William James, in address at least, and like him had countless admirers. Incidentally, he sponsored the James-Lange Theory of Emotions, and belongs to the functional-motor school in psychology, with a biological slant.

The Institut Jean-Jacques Rousseau, which he founded at the University of Geneva, in 1912, attracted many students from abroad who wanted to combine educational theory with experimental pedagogy.

JEAN PIAGET (1896—)

Jean Piaget, the successor of Flournoy and Claparède, at the University of Geneva, is one of the few living and probably the youngest of the investigators to be sketched in this volume, but that is because, being a prodigy, he matured so early.

As a lad he became engrossed in nature study, collecting molluscs and writing articles in a journal of zoology. By the age of eighteen, he had read dozens of books in philosophy and psychology. At the age of twenty, he published a philosophical novel. His doctorate was obtained in science at the University of Neuchâtel, with a thesis on molluscs. Zoology, geology, embryology, physical chemistry, and mathematics were his constant fare. It was not until 1918 that he left for greater adventure, settling in Zürich, where he worked in Lipps's laboratory and with Eugen Bleuler, the psychiatrist. He also attended lectures by Jung and Pfister, thus becoming inoculated with psychoanalytic doctrine.

Later at the Sorbonne, in Paris, he made various contacts with the important faculty men, among them Dr. Simon, who was Binet's collaborator in the standardization of the famous tests. He was put to the task of administering Binet's reading tests on Parisian children. Indifferent at first, he soon recognized that he had found his particular field; and his new enthusiasm was to probe into the failures of children rather than merely classify them on the basis of their successes. He discovered, for instance, that children up to the age of eleven or twelve experienced difficulties in reasoning unsuspected by adults. He supplemented his findings with results gained with abnormal children at La Salpêtrière and began to publish his articles in the *Journal de Psychologie* (Paris) and in Claparède's *Archives de Psychologie* (Geneva). On the basis of his first article, Claparède offered the author the post of director of studies at the J. J. Rousseau Institute.

Piaget, an industrious worker, has since brought out more than a score of books, the most important of which deal with the reasoning processes in children. It is a far cry from molluscs to children, yet a common basis can be found in Piaget's approach. The relationship of part to whole was the dominant problem. "The child can grasp a certain operation only if he is capable, at the same time, of correlating operations by modifying them in different well-determined ways—for instance, by inverting them." The detours or reversible steps depend, be believes, on groupings.

Piaget's conclusions have been challenged in the United States as too loaded with assumptions, e.g., that children are philosophical reasoners and that there are age zones where changes occur abruptly at the borderlines.

H

SCANDINAVIAN PSYCHOLOGY (Denmark)

HARALD HOEFFDING (1843-1931)

Harald Høffding was more a philosopher than a psychologist, known principally for his two-volume *History of Philosophy* but since he was of the *avant-garde* in Scandinavian psychology, having published his textbook, in Danish, as early as 1882, we cannot afford to omit him from our purview.

Unlike the Italian psychologists, who were good physiologists, Høffding was steeped in the humanities, particularly in philosophy. Kierkegaard, no doubt, exercised quite an influence on him, and his lasting interest in the psychology of religion is possibly the result of this.

Høffding was a critical observer. No experimentalist, he wrote books on thought, humor, experience and interpretation (somewhat in the vein of James's *Varieties of Religious Experience*), and dabbled in psychic research. His attitude toward behaviorism and, indeed, any physicalistic interpretation of mind was negative.

Regarded as one of the intellectual greats in Denmark, he was accorded royal honors and presented with a palatial home. A dominating personality, he succeeded in keeping his equally famous rival, Georg (Cohen) Brandes from the successful pursuit of an academic career.

ALFRED LEHMANN (1858-1921)

It was Alfred Lehmann who may be regarded as the first true Danish psychologist. At Leipzig, under Wundt, he had worked on the pulse and breathing curves, in line with Wundt's theories. These expressive methods, pioneered by Mosso at the University of Turin, were the rage around the turn of the century because they were supposed to neatly correlate physiological with psychological processes. In 1892, appeared the German translation of his important Danish work, *Fundamental Laws of Human Affective Life.*

Lehmann was a careful experimenter, not the type forever bubbling with new ideas and projects. As director of the laboratory which he founded at the University of Copenhagen, he enjoyed the respect of the many students he trained in the painstaking procedures of the newer techniques.

Edgar Rubin, as we have already seen under another rubric (Gestalt) was Director of the Psychological Laboratory at Copenhagen, Anathon Aal was the best-known psychologist in Norway. Martin L. Reymert, who had settled in the United States, where he was active until shortly before his death in 1953, made his first contribution in Norway. In Finland, A. Grotenfeld's name appears to have been widely recognized.

I
PILLARS OF RUSSIAN PSYCHOLOGY

IVAN PETROVICH PAVLOV (1848-1936)
Founder of Reflexology

The greatest name in Russian physiology, which has influenced all the mental sciences, is that of Pavlov. After graduating from the Military Academy in St. Petersburg Pavlov taught there and later studied under Ludwig and Heidenhain, two of the most eminent men in the field, in Germany.

His famous experiments on conditioned reflexes in dogs, revealing much new information on the process of digestion, earned him the Nobel Prize in 1904.

The familiar diagram of the dog drooling saliva in measurable quantities not only at the sight of food, but at the sound of a bell which was formerly sounded when the dog was fed became a stand-by in psychology textbooks. The experiments were supposed to demonstrate that no process of mental association was needed to produce such responses, but that it took place on an unconscious level, like digestion itself; on the other hand, there was no proof that association did not enter.

Pavlov's reflexology became the psychophysiological gospel in all USSR institutions of learning, although the originator himself was far from committing himself to a purely materialistic philosophy. Indeed, he was opposed to Communism, but living at a time when Lenin was the ruler and Stalin had not yet engaged in his ruthless purges, Pavlov enjoyed his freedom and remained an ornament in Communist science as under the Czarist regime.

Pavlov admittedly owed much to the founder of Russian physiology, J. M. Sechenov, whose *Reflexes of the Brain,* published in 1863, influenced the young aspirant immensely. Particularly was he impressed by Sechenov's laboratory discovery of central inhibition, which was a landmark at that time.

It has been urged by popular writers that the practice of brainwashing, the wresting of confessions from political victims, and, in general, the molding of the Russian masses have been achieved through Pavlovian principles. As a matter of fact, all education and, by the same token, all demoralization proceeded along similar lines, long before there was a Russia; and humans have been treated like dogs from time immemorial.

Actually, Pavlov belonged philosophically and psychologically to the school of Huxley and the epiphenomenalists. He can scarcely be called a materialist, let alone a dialectic materialist. He believed that mind was simply analogous to the sound of the bell or the spark which functions only at given times, when the physical (physiological) processes are adequately set up.

It is not generally known that Pavlov was born into the family of a Russian priest, and that he received his secondary education at a theological seminary "which I recall with gratitude."

In his short autobiographical sketch, he tells us: "I have renounced practicality in life with its cunning and not always irreproachable ways and I see no reason for regretting this; on the contrary, precisely in this do I find more certain consolation."

That Pavlov was a very scrupulous and unassuming person is evident from the fact that in his last days and after a serious operation, he took the trouble to send a note to the present writer to tell him that he must of necessity decline the invitation to participate in a *Festschrift,* honoring Freud on his eightieth birthday.

VLADIMIR BEKHTEREV (1857-1927)

Along with Pavlov, Bekhterev takes rank as Russia's leading physiologist, but because of his elder colleague's fame as a Nobel Prize laureate and his experiments on the conditioned reflex, Bekhterev has been overshadowed by him.

Bekhterev, after spending years in investigating the localization of brain functions, turned to neuropathology as his chief field. He was the first to describe a disease which was named for him, viz., the hardening of the spine from top to bottom in aged people, who yet can fully move their shoulders and hips. He described in detail several brain centers and fibers.

Better trained than Pavlov, he studied with Wundt and Flechsig at the University of Leipzig, and with Charcot in Paris; and in 1885, he was appointed to a professorship at the University of Kazan. In 1893, he took Merzheyevsky's post at the University of St. Petersburg, founding the first psychoneurological Institute in Russia (later changed to Psychoneurological Academy). He was the founder of various journals and societies, and his books on neurology have earned him wide recognition beyond the Russian borders.

Like Pavlov, he was a reflexologist. Physiology and neurology were the common denominator for both, but while Pavlov worked on dogs, and therefore the human equation had for him only a marginal interest, Bekhterev, as a psychiatrist, came face to face with human problems every day, and he was more sociopolitically involved than Pavlov.

Nevertheless, Bekhterev could be labeled a behaviorist. He himself preferred the designation "objective psychologist." According to him, "the object of psychoreflexology is the study of the relation of the organism to the external world in connection with the occurring experience, quite independent of the subjective experience."

That Bekhterev could not abandon the higher mental processes in his psychological system is evident from the fact that he tried to bridge the gap between ordinary reflexes and such operations as volition by introducing the term "personal reflexes," which is almost a reversal of his original position.

J

AMERICAN PSYCHOLOGY

Psychology was known and taught at Harvard under the aegis of physics from around 1640, although it was then called "pneumatics." Samples of propositions which had to be defended by students are:

A vehement sensation destroys the sense.
One Body does not House a Plurality of Souls.
The first things known consists of a single substance.
Life is the Union of Form and Substance.

All subjects were taught out of Latin textbooks, and the theses were supported in Latin.

It almost goes without saying that all observations, deduced by scholastic methods, had to conform to theological dogma. Fact was subservient to theory, and theorizing was invariably in the interest of theism. The "pneuma" or "breath" was merely the physical approach to the soul—a concession to physics, or, as it was then called, natural philosophy.

COTTON MATHER (1663-1728)

Until the rise of Cotton Mather, such psychologists as there were in New England were anonymous. Nor would Mather be recognized as such in our sense of the word. The fact, however, that he delivered himself of a number of observations bearing on the mind-body relationship, and that he included a chapter on melancholy in his theologico-medical treatise labeled "*The Angel of Bethesda,*" entitles him to be considered the first articulate American psychologist.

What has now become the fashion, namely, to combine the pastoral with the healing function, was actually practiced by Mather, who had wavered between the medical profession and the ministry, and while he eventually decided upon the latter, he had meanwhile done a good deal of medical reading, which constituted the major part of the medical training of the time.

Like most clergymen of his day, and some well-known medical men of a later generation (like Heinroth, in Germany), Mather believed that the cause of disease was sin, ever reverting to the first sin of the original human couple. The first step toward cure, then, was for the sinner-patient to become a penitent, but clergyman-semi-physician Mather also prescribed formulae from the famous Sydenham, from old wives' empiricals, and his own concoctions. He seemed to be more concerned with smallpox and fever than with anything else. Most of the remedies were either harmless or mildly prescribed, i.e., with certain reservations. He knew of germs or insect animalcula, as he refers to them, and apparently browsed in the medical literature of the day. "Mercury," he declaims, "We know thee, but we are afraid, that thou wilt kill us too, if we employ thee to kill them that kill us." His shrewd aperçus are, of course, often vitiated by the meager information of the day. Nevertheless he concludes that the body being a machine, the physician should understand "the natural organization, structure and operations of the machine which he undertakes to regulate."

A Puritan divine, such as Mather was, would naturally look to the Hebrew Bible for his first principles. Thus it is that he harps on the phrase "*nishmath-chajim*" ("khayim," it should be), which to him may be of a "middle nature, between the rational soul and the corporeal mass . . . the medium of communication by which they work upon one another. It wonderfully receives also impressions from both of them." The "*nishmath khayim*" which Mather rides so persistently is evidently the origin of our "animal spirits." In Jewish lore, it is simply the soul of man, no connecting link ("*neshamah*" is the word—"*nishmath*" is the construct form, with the implication of "of").

Since Mather takes sin to be the cause of sickness of the spirit, which in turn will lead to bodily disease, what about the "insects" and "animalcula" which invade our bodies? I suppose that Mather might retort that unless our spirit were run down, the invaders would have no chance of surviving.

Mather found bodily ailments to designate each of the vices. Thus lust is a distemper of the soul; an unsteady soul has a palsy; a wanton soul has a fever, a worldly soul has a dropsy; while anger is likened to erysipelas, envy rather extremely to cancer, and sloth to scurvy. (Capsula 1, in *The Angel of Bethesda*)

"Melancholy" is the theme of Chapter XXV of the *Angel of Bethesda.* In brief compass, he gives the healer some solitary advice within a theological framework. He tells what others have prescribed: a bag of saffron worn over the heart, and a drink of whey, infused with epithymum. He warns against charms and incantations, which, for one who was partly instrumental in the hanging of "witches," would mean entering into traffic with the Devil.

SAMUEL JOHNSON (1696-1772)—
The First Psychological Author in America

If Cotton Mather was the first known writer to incorporate psychological discussions in his works, Samuel Johnson, also a clergyman, might be regarded as the first to give us a compendium of psychology, derived largely from Locke's *Essay*, but tinged with theological dogma.

Precocious to the extent of compiling a diminutive encyclopedia at the age of nineteen, he subsequently became the first President of King's College, later Columbia University. Possessed of a charming address, he ably executed the various functions of college president, teacher, and textbook author, as well as those of a preacher.

Naturally psychology is still called "pneumatology," for Johnson still clings to the "soul" as the *fons et origo* of the mental operations. It is the soul which is the source of the *retention* of an idea, as it is the power "whereby after the disappearing of an idea, it can recollect and call it to mind again." Sometimes he is more explicit than Locke, and in his definition of perception, he makes sure to say that ideas are nothing but actual perceptions, which cease to be anything when there is no perception of them, but later, after making the acquaintance of Berkeley, he was to embrace the Irish Bishop's spiritual idealism.

For his period, Samuel Johnson followed a liberal course, even if he explains all our knowledge as due to the "universal presence and action of the Deity." He could perceive a distinction between *memory* and *remembrance,* between *attention* and *intention,* and he employs the term "apprehension" (which Locke avoids) to designate the process of perception.

JONATHAN EDWARDS (1703-1758)—
The Fiery Preacher

In a sense, the high-strung, impetuous Jonathan Edwards can be contrasted with the urbane and versatile Samuel Johnson. Entering Yale at thirteen, and becoming a tutor there at twenty-three, he left the academic sphere to become a pastor at Northampton, where he preached his fire-and-brimstone sermons to a terrified community, for practically all of the adult inhabitants were communicants. This crusader championed certain tenets which were too extreme even for the zealous of the eighteenth century, and soon he was driven from his parish, living as a missionary among the Indians at Stockbridge, Massachusetts. Here he wrote his famous *Inquiry into the Freedom of the Will* and *The Affections,* which may be regarded as the first independent works in psychology by an American.

Jonathan Edwards stands out as probably the most colorful personality in early American theology and philosophy. He is generally rated as the most important thinker in the Colonies prior to the Revolution. A subtle dialectician and an incisive publicist, he was able to whip up the imagination of his listeners through effective illustrations and powerful rhetoric.

What a paradox that this gaunt apostle of determinism, who expostulated away the freedom of the will, was himself possessed of an indomitable will that no opponent could crush. And what an irony that this fanatical St. Bernard of a later era should have propagated a psychological doctrine which coincided with those of the materialist, Hobbes, and the non-theist, Spinoza! But while the two great philosophers were content to rest their case after proving that we are not free to will, Edwards takes us a step farther, insisting that all human choice is, in reality, rooted in the will of God. In the last analysis, Edwards says that we are free to choose what we desire at a given moment, but, alas, *our desiring is not of our choice.*

Edwards wrote ten books, which enjoyed several editions, but his personality and influence interest us perhaps even more than his works. He was constantly at loggerheads with the more moderate leaders of the community and he certainly was not a favorite of the gods. At one time he led a precarious existence which necessitated the selling of homemade laces at fairs, and after losing two highly regarded sons-in-law, he himself died at the age of fifty-five, about a month before he was to assume the duties of President of Princeton College, in replacement of his deceased son-in-law. His numerous descendants of high distinction have become a standard argument in favor of the genetic (heredity) conception as against the theory of total environmentalism.

Hysterical Phenomena

Jonathan Edwards was not only a theoretical psychologist. He also produced psychological phenomena of some consequence; and he was the first in America to probe the state of mind of those who had fallen under his spell.

In New England, hysteria and other neurotic tendencies were probably more rampant than in other regions. The hanging of "witches" in Salem affords us an illustration which is not paralleled elsewhere in this country. We can well imagine how the brooding members of Edwards' parish would react to the furious castigations of their pastor—the lurid pictures of the Devil, the horrible descriptions of what awaits sinners in hell. Small wonder that the mentally depressed became desperate, and occasionally someone tried suicide. Edwards naturally set himself up as a therapist; but strange to say, his results were not always successful. Instead of being calmed, some who, in his words "seemed to be under no melancholy . . . nor were under any special trouble or concern of mind about anything spiritual or temporal, yet had it urged upon them, as if somebody had spoken to them *"Cut your throat, now is a good opportunity!"*

As might be expected, Edwards attributed his success to God, his failures to the Devil, but the studies which he made of specific cases throw light on the subject of individual differences, so that we have here a pioneer in a field which was to be cultivated only centuries later.

We have mentioned that this religious zealot defended a thesis held by Hobbes and Spinoza. Perhaps more remarkable is the fact that in his sermon, "Men Naturally God's Enemies," he seems to approach Freud's view that the father is hated as the symbol of authority, and in prehistoric times was killed by the sons, and that there is a mass tendency to kill a leader. Edwards maintained that the reason his communicants were not conscious of their desire to kill God was its sheer impossibility—"But if the life of God were within your reach and you knew it, it would not be safe one hour." The continuity of man in God's action—since, according to Edwards, we are all guilty because of Adam's sin—has its analogy in Freud's theory of recurrence—strange points of contact!

S. S. SMITH (1750-1819)— The First Environmentalist Thinker

In Samuel Stanhope Smith, who succeeded his father-in-law, John Witherspoon, as President of the College of New Jersey (now Princeton), we have the first environmentalist, who sought causes for trait differences in climate, milieu, local needs, etc. Thus, he may be looked upon as a sociologist offering more or less original theories about certain characteristics in men and animals. "Out of the same strain the Pennsylvania Dutch raised large and heavy horses while the Irish bred a lighter and smaller animal, and horses will be black, white or bay, in accordance with the fashion of the day by choosing horses of the desired color to supply the studs."

Smith was an analyst of the Scottish Common Sense School, who laid less stress, however, on the inborn nature of man.

His remarks on assimilation in a country like the United States adumbrate the anthropological researches of Franz Boas, and his explanation of the kinky hair of Negroes in Africa seems plausible. He adds that "this conjecture received some confirmation by observing that the negroes born in the United States of America are gradually losing their strong smell of the African Zone; their hair is at the same time growing less involved and becoming denser and longer." We may gather that Smith in no wise thought the Negro to be inherently inferior, but rather the product of torrid climatic conditions. "It is well known," he writes, "that the Africans who have been brought to America are daily becoming, under all the disadvantages of servitude, more ingenious and susceptible of instruction." Bear in mind, also, that this little-known essay on the "causes of the variety of human complexion and figure" was composed about seventy-five years before the emancipation of the Negroes.

The First Definitive Textbook

Since early colonial days, textbooks of a sort had been published, most of them restricting psychology to one section of the work, which would be a compendium of metaphysics, theology, ethics, and "pneumatology." It was not, however, until 1827, that the first comprehensive psychological textbook appeared, under the title of *Elements of Intellectual Philosophy.* Four years later it was expanded into two volumes, titled *Elements of Mental Philosophy.* Slight as the change may seem, the substitution of the term "mental" for "intellectual" is a sign of progress. The author, Thomas C. Upham (1789-1872), like so many of his predecessors, was a clergyman who taught philosophy (Bowdoin College), and it was no slight distinction that his American textbook was used extensively in England. In this country, edition after edition appeared, and even as late as 1886, fourteen years after the author's death, a new printing was called for.

Upham's work was noted for its breadth, its systematic coverage, its plethora of apt illustrations from biography, travel, history and fiction, and its smooth style, reminiscent of Thomas Brown's. One of its most appealing features is a clarity which had been rare among the theological authors who preceded him.

His analysis of the emotions and the sentiments, in

all their nuances, is almost as keen as McDougall's, a century later, and in a few instances, he foreshadows principles that came to light subsequently. When he digresses into sociological territory, dealing with mass behavior—*e.g.*, statistics relating to mail, financial estimates, and crime—he comes close to the reasoning of Buckle and his materialistic conception of history. "All things conclusively evince," says Upham, "that the actions of men, whether considered individually or in masses, are not placed beyond the reach of some forms of law, and are not left to mere chance or accident." Today this seems commonplace, but not 130 years ago.

It must also be mentioned that Upham was the first to devote considerable space in his works to a description of abnormal behavior and phenomena, with more than a modicum of sound counsel, not based on religious admonition.

German Immigrant First to Use Psychology Label

One of the most remarkable pioneers in the field was Frederick Augustus Rauch (1806-1841), who while still in his twenties was slated for the chair in metaphysics at the University of Heidelberg, when his expression of solidarity with the fraternities opposing the government made it necessary for him to seek employment in the United States.

At first he taught music and German at Lafayette College, then qualified for the ministry and became professor in Biblical literature at the German Reformed Theological Seminary at York, Pennsylvania. Later, he organized Marshall College, and became its first president. This checkered career lay behind a man of thirty. Only half of the Biblical span of life was reserved for him, and a year before his untimely death, appeared his *Psychology or a View of the Human Soul, including Anthropology,* which was exhausted a few weeks after its publication. A second edition came out shortly after his death, in 1841.

Why was this young man a pioneer? In the first place, he discarded the hackneyed terms "intellectual" and "mental" philosophy. Then, he made the first attempt to blend German and American thought, not merely citing a passage here and there from Kant. What he calls "anthropology," after the Kantian fashion, is the material which relates to the individual in the light of his environment: sex differences, national characteristics, temperament, sleep and dreams—in other words much of what goes into our textbooks. Psychology as it was then understood in Germany belonged to a higher sphere—the more complex mental states and processes.

Rauch may be considered the first personalist in America—perhaps anywhere. "The person is not only the centre of man, but also the centre of nature." While he often speaks in metaphors, and some psychological terms are used loosely (e.g., "perception" instead of "idea"), perhaps the result of his inability to rid himself of his early German training, he was, in a sense, a trail blazer. His reflections on semantics place him in the ranks of pioneers in that field as well.

First Objectivist in America

Those who believe that John B. Watson was the first behaviorist will probably be surprised to learn that James Rush (1786-1869), brilliant son of the pioneer in American psychiatry, was the iconoclast who first parted company with those psychologists who built on a religious foundation, more than a century ago.

Evidently a prodigy, he went to study at the University of Edinburgh with the representatives of the Scottish School, but those early studies left him wholly dissatisfied. After returning to the United States, he launched upon a laborious investigation of the human voice, which was completed in 1827. But as Rush wished not only to inaugurate a new method in teaching voice, based on his independent theories, but to introduce a complicated terminology of his own, including a radically simplified spelling ("impune" for "impugn," "plaines" for "plainness," "thot" for "thought"), no publisher would take the risk of bringing out his work. He had it printed at his own expense, and lived to revise the seventh enlarged edition. As a system of vocal training, it has had many adaptations.

What is of more concern to us here is his complete break with the traditional views of psychology, his stress on the speech organs and on the muscles in general. In other words, *motor theories begin with Rush.* Nearly a century ago, he held that *the mind consisted not only of perceiving and thinking but also of speaking and acting.*

In the two volumes constituting his *Brief* (sic) *Outline of an Analysis of the Human Intellect Intended to rectify the scholastic and vulgar perversions of the natural purpose and method of thinking; by rejecting altogether the theoretic confusion, the unmeaning arrangement and indefinite nomenclature of the metaphysician,* he frankly espouses a materialistic position. Likening the brain to a reflecting mirror, he answers the question whether matter can think by changing the term "think" to "reflect" and contending that "an image and type [type is to Rush a non-visual image] being made on the matter of the brain must by reciprocity of action be material." He is ready to wait for strict demonstration by means of the microscope or other physical instrument, but so far as he is concerned, the *images are not only the proximate cause of thought but are thought itself.*

Like Watson, more than half a century later, he advocated the study of animal behavior, and like him, he would now and then belabor the psychologists of the day, who "without a speck of analogy, hanging on some antiquated authority of Gods and men, believe they have the demonstrated fact of spirit."

Small wonder that James Rush, never pulling his punches, and antagonizing all the academic psychologists, at a time when the clergy held the fort and an iconoclast like himself would be regarded as a crackpot (especially when he chose to present his views in what they thought an erratic form)—small wonder he was ignored and forgotten, despite his many novel ideas and astute remarks on various types of people, professions, and national groups.

Like his father, James Rush championed unpopular causes, but he did not possess Benjamin's social graces, his extraverted nature, and his sense of compromise. Hence, despite his acumen and incisive writing, and his prepossessing appearance, instead of mellowing in advanced age, he became dour and embittered.

Hickock—The Methodologist

Were it not for the fact that with all his theological leanings, Laurens P. Hickock (1798-1888) had some modern insights and that he appears to be the foremost dialectician of the period, he would not be assigned a place in this historical survey.

The author of a 700-page volume of *Rational Psychology* (1848) and a smaller *Empirical Psychology* (1854), he is primarily a methodologist in his differentiation between rational psychology—which he maintains to be more fundamental and which should enable us to make psychology an exact science—and empirical psychology, which can only give us results of a fragmentary nature. Hickock is concerned with the *rationale* of the experience, not with the experience as such.

Some of the problems he discussed were later grappled with, on a higher level, by James and others, but it was he who employed, in the psychological sense, probably for the first time the terms *introspection, psychographic,* and *conditioned.* His twofold division of psychology, coming down to us from the Scholastics, has had its counterparts in all periods, whether in act and existential psychologies or in purposive and causal psychologies.

Porter and McCosh

The two men who played the most important part in American psychology just prior to the scientific era which began with William James, are Noah Porter (1811-1892), President of Yale, and James McCosh (1811-1894), President of Princeton. Both may have been overrated in their day because of the influence they wielded as able administrators, but their widely used textbooks contained much thoughtful material, ably expounded.

Both men were dominating personalities. Porter banned Spencer's *Principles of Sociology* at Yale, but McCosh, the last of the Scottish Mohicans, was more adaptable in that he favored the doctrine of evolution. Porter wielded a trenchant pen in his attempt to confound the more liberal thinkers of his time. McCosh was less encyclopedic in his range, but his approach to topics was more factual. He was probably the first to introduce pictorial material, actually crudely drawn figures, in a psychological textbook published in this country. McCosh lived long enough to review James's *Principles of Psychology,* which he thought too mechanistic. McCosh's best textbook is that on the emotions (1880), which retains a certain value even today, thanks to its plenitude of keen insights.

John Dewey

John Dewey (1859-1952) ranks as one of the foremost philosophers in America. In some quarters, he is even rated above William James, but his influence in psychology was largely indirect; for although he was probably the first in the United States to speak of the "new psychology" and to set forth its aims at the age of twenty-five, and even published a textbook in his twenties, it was as a professor of philosophy that he served all his life, first at the University of Michigan, then at the University of Chicago, and subsequently at Columbia.

Nevertheless his influence was considerable. It seemed at first that he had departed from the religious implications of the clergymen-psychologists. Yet, in his 427-page *Psychology,* written when he was twenty-seven or twenty-eight, he speaks of the "reaction of the soul upon a nervous impulse" and states that "every concrete act of knowledge involves an intuition of God." The young man from the hills of Vermont delves into the specific problems of psychology, and shows signs of veering from the beaten path, even in his earliest articles, "The Psychological Standpoint" and "Psychology as a Philosophic Method."

In his very first published article, where he outlines the differences between the old and the new psychologies, we are struck with the use of a phrase which began to take on its proper significance only decades later. That phrase is "dynamic psychology," which he contrasts with what he called "psychostatics." The "new psychology," he asserts, "believes that truth, that reality, not necessarily *beliefs about reality,* is given in the living experience of the soul's development."

Germ of Functionalism

Despite his use of theological concepts, he manages to blaze new paths, revealing the seed of instrumentalism in philosophy and of functionalism in psychology, when, e.g., he considers the "idea of environment as a necessity to the idea of organism," and is critical of a view which treats the individual as an isolated thing in a vacuum. He thus provides the science with a new frame of reference—the relationship of individual to environment.

At the University of Chicago, where he remained for a decade, he had under his tutelage J. R. Angell, who before becoming President of Yale, led the functionalist revolt in psychology; and the Chicago group became the opponents of Cornell and its giant, E. B. Titchener, who taught an ingrown elementarism, without considering combinations and coordinations. An article that made a stir in its day was Dewey's "The Reflex Arc Concept in Psychology" (1896), which suggested that the reflex arc, and not the nerve cell or impulse, was the elementary unit, after which *larger* and more elaborate co-ordinations followed, each in its own partial function making for some objective end.

Titchener, an Englishman trained at Oxford and Leipzig, was ready to build up his psychology out of sensations, images, ideas, emotions, etc.—the contents of consciousness, regardless of purposes or practical aims. Dewey, the typical American, was not satisfied with such a sterile structure. To him anything which happens must answer some need or goal. The functional view is biologically colored, and is, therefore, more practical than a purely scientific construction; and the practical project will always get the upper hand in any kind of human endeavor. From the very beginning, John Dewey took up the attitude that psychology must be of aid in other human spheres. When he was thirty, he and J. A. McLellan brought out a book on "Applied Psychology," but it dealt wholly with the principles and practice of education; and it was this domain that Dewey virtually dominated for half a century. Progressive education is largely of his making; and only now is it beginning to be apparent that the pendulum which he started moving had gone altogether too far in the other direction. As a famed professor in America's largest university, he could affect the educational systems of remote countries through the thousands of foreign students who absorbed his teachings, but in his own land, too, he was accepted as a prophet.

THE SCIENTIFIC ERA IN AMERICAN PSYCHOLOGY

WILLIAM JAMES, Foremost American Psychologist

If the younger Dewey precedes the older James (1842-1910) in these pages, it is only because his textbook antedated the classic work of William James, who took almost a decade to complete his *magnum opus*. Once it appeared, in 1890, in two volumes containing about 1500 pages, it was immediately recognized as the greatest psychological textbook, at least in English, that had thus far come off the press. Not that it was acclaimed universally. The clergymen-psychologists certainly could not swallow James's tenets, wholly unencumbered by theological implications. The Germans, again, balked at the unsystematic presentation of topics, at its rambling and sprawling utterances, which were just what added flavor to what, under other circumstances, might have been a dry and dull treatise.

Suffice it to say that the freshness of the point of view, the masterly treatment of the main issues, the introduction of human-interest illustrations, the authority manifest in the handling of scientific data—whether they belonged to chemistry, physiology, or anatomy—and lastly, the inimitable style must have struck the initiates as well as the instructors as something of an entirely different order from what they had been accustomed to read.

Whether it was James or Wundt who opened the first psychological laboratory does not really much matter. There is hardly an idea or principle which emanated directly and independently from him, as in the case of Fechner, Helmholtz, Hering, and Lotze. Yet he deserved his laurels as a first-rate psychologist, who brought to his science a vast fund of data and, what is even more valuable, an *understanding of human nature.* There was greater immediacy in his approach than in that of Wundt, who trudged along experimentally and built up his science systematically and yet the resultant structure stood bare.

> James's range or scope was not nearly so extensive as Wundt's, but there was great sweep and penetration for specific sectors of knowledge, and, of course, a greater understanding of human nature from the inside, as immediacy and not merely as scientific constructs. Wundt would trudge on and on with blinders on his eyes, and would not budge to look around, lest he stray from the beaten path. James, on the other hand, would get into a trotting pace, ever on the alert for some casual event which, although it might slow him up a bit and even divert him, would nevertheless bear on the purpose of his journey. While Wundt would move in a rectilinear direction, and would turn at right angles only after a definite lap had been completed, James did not hesitate to roam about and even retrace his steps, or go back and forth, in order to make sure that he was not taking the wrong road after all.
>
> William James was the Midas of mind. Everything he touched, or rather experienced, was turned into psychic gold. What the world would frown upon as undesirable, or even a failure, James could turn to good account.[6]

James's Celtic ancestry and early environment must have had something to do with his shift of interest, with his conflict between artistic and scientific inclinations, and with the fact that his *Principles of Psychology* was not completed until he was nearly fifty, after he had embarked upon various careers (art, engineering, medicine) which ended in his teaching anatomy and physiology at the Harvard Medical School. Thence he advanced to psychology and finally to philosophy, where his name is associated with radical empiricism and pragmatism.

In psychology, he affiliated himself more with the French school than with the German. The clinical case, the deviate, the possible exception, engaged his ear and eye. This explains why he gave us his *Varieties of Religious Experience*, why he engaged in psychic research. It is why he formulated the organic theory of emotions—or, as it is generally known, the James-Lange theory—according to which there is nothing mental about an emotion, only the awareness of what is going on in the blood vessels and the internal organs, when we perceive something to frighten or anger us and we are set to run or fight, so that the order of events is the reverse of what we generally hold. Thus, we hear an explosion, and we run, which causes us to undergo certain *physiological changes* that mean fright. We feel sorry because we cry and not the other way around. This hypothesis received much discussion, but proved too vulnerable to become accepted.

Perhaps James's greatest assets were his gracious and benign personality, his social intelligence, and his charm. Wherever he traveled, he made a host of friends, and these soon became, if not his disciples, at least high-grade press agents. In terms of productivity his achievement was not great, but whatever he did write was backed by authority, even if the issue as a whole was controversial.

He believed in free will, which was not according to psychological Hoyle, and held other "unorthodox" views. But he may have been induced to take up such positions for practical purposes, just as Kant, after disposing of the regulative ideas in his *Critique of Pure Reason,* embraced them in his *Critique of Practical Reason,* since an ethical life loses its prop and validity without the acceptance of certain assumptions. Even the motor theory of consciousness which James taught had its practical consideration. Mooning, brooding without an outlet, bodes no good. Conversion into action was James's salutary advice.

STANLEY HALL and HIS RECORD OF FIRSTS

Granville Stanley Hall (1844-1924) was born on a farm at Ashfield, a village near Boston, but American psychology and education would have lost a precious organizer if this farm boy had remained in the ministry after graduation from the Union Theological Seminary. He was preparing to go to Leipzig, the Mecca of American graduate students in psychology, when he was offered a minor teaching post at Harvard, where he was able to carry some graduate work under James and Bowen.

He was the first to receive the Ph.D. in philosophy at Harvard University, at thirty-four, but before long, he chalked up for himself a record of firsts that would be the envy of any ambitious man. He was the first American student at the first officially accepted psychological laboratory during its first year of existence. He was the first to found a specifically psychological laboratory in the United States at Johns Hopkins (James's laboratory was functioning under the aegis of physiology). He launched the first psychological journal in the English language—*The American Journal of Psychology*. He was the first President of Clark University (1888), and he was the first President of the American Psychological Association, which he virtually organized.

Other journals which he founded were *The Pedagogical Seminary, The Journal of Genetic Psychology,* and the *Journal of Applied Psychology,* which are still in existence. Some journals which he started were discontinued after a number of years. Administering a new and growing university, with an expanding psychology department which required his direction and teaching, as well as editing several periodicals, involving a vast amount of correspondence, must have required the expenditure of tremendous energy, but it also required an outlay of thousands of dollars when his chief sponsor, expecting *The American Journal of Psychology* to be devoted mainly to psychic research, withdrew his backing. Hall was a man of vision and maintained his independence throughout life. He could very well have posed for a statue of a Minute Man, or a Civil War general. At both Johns Hopkins and Clark his students were much attached to him, although among his peers, he did not receive the homage which James or, later, Titchener received.

It was the field of genetic psychology that Stanley Hall cultivated chiefly. His students were assigned problems in child psychology, learning, adolescent activities, etc., while his large volumes on adolescence and senescence were much used works of reference by educators. The questionnaire as a method in psychology was largely devised by him. It was pooh-poohed by most of his colleagues, but it stood the test, and was the basis of Woodworth's Personal Data sheet and the form sent out to draftees during the first World War.

His journals were filled with articles on topics not dealt with in the laboratories—envy, anger, proverbs in a psychological light, fear.

GEORGE T. LADD—Last of the Church Mohicans

Born in the same year as William James, George T. Ladd (1842-1920) belongs to the prescientific group of preacher-psychologists, yet his *Elements of Physiological Psychology,* which preceded James' *Principles of Psychology* and became one of the most widely used and valued textbooks, served to give the author a scientific prestige. Like Stanley Hall who had wavered between joining the clergy and teaching psychology, Ladd, was interested in religious phenomena, in the person of Jesus. While he approached this sphere as an investigator, Ladd, like McCosh and the line which led up to him, sought the ultimate; and of his divided loyalty, psychology received the lesser share.

Ladd, who was graduated from Bowdoin, was appointed to the chair in philosophy at Yale in 1881, and in 1892, the year both Münsterberg and Titchener came to the United States, he founded the Yale Psychological Laboratory, later putting E. W. Scripture in charge. Ladd must have experienced a sore disappointment when Scripture left Yale under the shadow of an unconventional episode.

Despite his delving into physiological psychology, Ladd gave priority to the mental or psychic, regarding James as a mechanist. To Ladd, psychology was not a natural science. Ladd was still the soul psychologist, or if we wish to be gracious, we might say he was a personalist. To him the permanent self, which is always functioning and adapting itself to the needs of the organism, is the core of psychology as well as its goal; and the *will,* which modern psychology has largely rejected, became for him the cornerstone in this whole structure.

Ladd's various textbooks in psychology were well written and reminiscent of the earlier compendia. As he advanced in age, his books took on a more religious coloring. Such titles as *What Can I Know?, What Ought I to Do?, What Should I Believe?, What May I Hope?* are symptomatic of the reversion to preaching, albeit on a high level. Small wonder, then, that even *The Elements of Physiological Psychology* did not keep his name fresh in the minds of psychologists who looked up to James, Hall, Titchener, Cattell, and Münsterberg, though Ladd was the second President of the American Psychological Association, preceding James. After Woodworth expanded the *Elements,* the work was associated chiefly with the younger man. The final revision retained so little of the early editions that Ladd's name was subsequently dropped altogether.

J. McKEEN CATTELL—First Professor of Psychology

Up to this time, psychology had been under the tutelage of philosophy. J. McKeen Cattell (1860-1944) became the first professor of psychology. Curiously enough, it was neither Harvard nor Yale, nor even Columbia University, which made the break, but the University of Pennsylvania, in Philadelphia. From there Cattell took the title to Columbia, where he trained a whole generation of brilliant men, who branched out in psychology (Thorndike, Woodworth), anthropology (Clark Wissler), and physiology (S. J. Franz). His pacifism or individualism brought him into conflict with President Nicholas Murray Butler, and terminated his teaching career, though he received a court award of $40,000 as compensation for the summary dismissal.

Cattell, the son of a college president, in addition to his native endowment, brought to his field a happy synthesis of German training, gained at Leipzig under Wundt, and British methodology, acquired through his association with Francis Galton—"the greatest man whom I have known"—father of eugenics, composite photography, biometrics, and imaginal typology.

It was probably from Galton that Cattell received his statistical impetus, so that he was the only psychologist in the early days of the science to insist on quantification, ratings, and rankings in the mental sphere. This impulse he transmitted to the most brilliant of his students, E. L. Thorndike.

As early as 1890, Cattell focused attention on the

project of testing mental functions. Correlation was his forte, and he later inaugurated a series of studies on American men of science. In fact, he was the initiator of the various directories of American scientists and educators, and the editor of several psychological journals, first with J. Mark Baldwin, and then alone.

As he went deeper into publishing, he became more of an organizer of science, and rose to the presidency of the American Psychological Association, the American Association for the Advancement of Science, and the International Congress of Psychology at Yale in 1929.

Cattell wrote no books. His papers and addresses fill only two sizable volumes, yet he did not fritter away his time. This was spent in a vast correspondence, in designing apparatus, editing and publishing, organizing, and in academic counsel halls. In other words, he was a directive force in American psychology; and something, too, of a seer.

Seventy years ago, he sensed what turn psychology would take in succeeding decades. He used the term "mental tests" before Binet, although his tests were in the line of individual differences, and he advocated, in short words, the word-reading method rather than sound-letter teaching in schools. His stress on methods and techniques and his espousal of the objective approach, although not to the exclusion of introspection, brought him closer to what is now called operationism. Through the founding of the Psychological Corporation in New York, with a large contribution of his own, he has earned the title of a pioneer in the standardization of applied psychology.

As early as 1904, in an address on "The Conceptions and Methods of Psychology," he foresaw the ramifications of the science as well as its interrelation with many other sciences. In opposition to Münsterberg, he maintained that "sciences are not immutable species, but developing organisms." Cattell's aim was to fit psychology into a growing system where the circumstances of competition and co-operation would disclose the results at any given time. In this sense, he was a pragmatist, not as to validity but in respect to its place in a scientific efflorescence.

"THE MOTOR MAN ON THE PSYCHOLOGICAL CAR"

It was the distinction of James Mark Baldwin (1861-1934) to have been the founder of two psychological laboratories (University of Toronto and Princeton) and the restorer of the Johns Hopkins Laboratory, which had fallen into disuse after Hall's departure to become President of Clark University. He was also the moving spirit of the four-volume *Dictionary of Philosophy and Psychology* (of which two constituted B. Rand's Bibliography), which he edited. He, furthermore, was co-editor and founder of several psychological periodicals, but unlike Cattell, with whom he collaborated for a time, he was a prolific author. When only twenty-nine, the first volume of his *Handbook of Psychology* came off the press, to be followed by *Mental Development in the Child and the Race* (1894), *Social and Ethical Interpretations* (1897), and his four-volume *Thought and Things or Genetic Logic* which brought him fame, especially in Europe, where he received many citations. Next to William James, he was the most translated American psychologist, and his election to a dozen learned societies afforded him a great deal of apparent gratification.

For all his service to psychological laboratories Baldwin was not a laboratory man, as was Cattell. Whether it was the influence of McCosh, or his own Scottish family tradition, he was not free from a certain theological bias, which culminated in his enrolling in the Princeton Theological Seminary. Mc-

Cosh advised his charge to make a trip to Germany, which did not impress him. In France, however, he made contacts with Charcot, Janet, and Bernheim, as well as with other noted men in the field. Apparently he lost his heart to France, for his views were more in harmony with the French school than with the German, the French stressing the affective as against the cognitive, the functional as against the structural in psychology. It was to France he retreated after a deplorable incident led to the termination of his academic career.

Baldwin's expatriate existence and the fact that, unlike Cattell, he had no group of influential students may account for his being forgotten as an important leader in the first decade of the century. Another reason is the philosophical and sociological texture of his works. In his psychology, there are three strains: (a) the genetic; (b) the functional; and (c) the social. He was a strong advocate of evolution and propounded a theory of organic selection according to which the *individual, through effort, is constantly learning to mold his natural inheritance.* Thus, the will becomes a paramount factor in his system. Overlooking the verbiage in some of his weightier books, there is much in them that was stimulating and even fresh for the time. His was a blend of the Scottish and the French—a balanced combination, with the philosophical leading the psychological. His erudition was immense and is apparent even in the two slender volumes on the *History of Psychology.* His own sketch happens to be the first in the series of psychological autobiographies which were begun in 1930 at Clark University.

Baldwin was a promoter, not only of psychology but of himself. He was an early sponsor of the motor theory of consciousness and that other great promoter, Hugo Münsterberg, once remarked to him, "You and I are the motor men on the psychological car."

E. B. TITCHENER, Psychological Ruler

Of all the sometime rulers in psychology, Edward Bradford Titchener (1867-1927) seems to have suffered the greatest neglect. Fifty years ago, his was a name to conjure with. Invited to Cornell, in 1892, after a thorough education at Oxford embracing the humanities, philosophy, and physiology, and a doctorate from Leipzig under Wundt, he soon made the Cornell laboratory a beehive of research, to which able graduate students flocked for experimental training in the expanding science. Many of Titchener's students became eminent psychologists, directors of laboratories in the United States and Canada and even abroad. In time, the Titchener experimentalists began to meet annually as a clan with special aspirations.

What is it that drew students to Titchener? In the first place, his air of self-assurance and bearded dignity, supported by a stately frame, his mastery of English and preparedness for all sorts of contingencies, his vast learning and readiness to burrow into such remote fields for the time as Russian or Arabic, his showmanship in the delivery of his lectures, and, of course, his critical and thoroughgoing manner of conducting research. Students who at times felt slighted knew that he had a fatherly feeling for them; and if he brooked no opposition in the laboratory, he was nevertheless ready to express his appreciation of accomplishment.

To some of his advanced students he became a

father image, which they tried to emulate. Fifty years ago he and Münsterberg, at Harvard, seemed to dominate American psychology, and while the latter got into the public eye through his popular appeal, Titchener rated as the true scientist, faithful to his goal.

Perhaps it would be apt here to quote from the man who turned out to be the ablest of his students, E. G. Boring:

> What a man! To me he has always seemed the nearest approach to genius of anyone with whom I have been closely associated. I used to watch my conversations with him, hoping I might gain some insight into why his thinking was so much better than mine. I decided presently that his superiority lay in his easy command of memory traces, his ready entertainment of novel relationships, his equally ready abandonment of unprofitable hypotheses, and his avidity in the pursuit of goals. His mind seemed never to gather wool, never to try the same blind alley twice. Titchener loved to solve puzzles, and his skill in numismatics was developed over the problems posed by Mohammedan coins. He was always ready with unexpected advice. If you had mushrooms, he would tell you how to cook them. If you were buying oak for a new floor, he would at once come forward with all the advantages of ash. If you were engaged to be married, he would have his certain and insistent advice about the most unexpected aspects of your problems, and, if you were honeymooning, he would write to remind you, as he did me, on what day you ought to be back at work. Seldom did he distinguish between his wisdom and his convictions and he never hid either.

The stories about Titchener are legion but this is not his biography. Most of the stories centered upon his personality—his dominance or his mag-

> netism, depending on how you regarded his contact with your life. Many of his more able graduate students came to resent his interference and control and eventually rebelled, to find themselves suddenly on the outside, excommunicated, bitter, with return impossible. Quite early in our married life my wife and I decided that we would accept "insults" and arbitrary control from Titchener in order to retain the stimulus and charm of his sometimes paternal and sometimes patronizing friendship. I never broke with the master and I still feel that the credit remained on my side.[7]

Boring never broke with him, but after the latter's death, he abandoned Titchener's systematic views and became an objectivist, a physicalist, and an operationist—everything which would have made Titchener turn over in his grave.

What was Titchener's psychology like? He was generally regarded as Wundt's apostle in America; for Titchener aimed at building up a system in which every phenomenon would be pigeonholed and related to some other phenomenon. He was a strict psychophysical parallelist, believing in the twin series of physiological and psychological processes, and above all a structuralist in that the edifice which we call the mind he believed built up of such elements as sensations, images, ideas, feelings. All the elements must be *in consciousness*. Hence, habit, action, instinct, and any Freudian mechanism received either marginal treatment from him, or none at all. Freudian complexes could not exist for him. If only the conscious is grist for the psychological mill, then the introspective method is the only one which can furnish the data. The phenomena might be explained later through physiology, but in his several textbooks, Titchener showed no alacrity to go into such explanations except for the very elementary sensory processes.

Titchener's laboratory manuals have never been

surpassed, but where the science has taken altogether different directions, the methods have necessarily become obsolete. And that was the tragedy of Titchener. He stuck to his Wundtian guns, remained the *pure* scientist, interested solely in general laws and discovering new phenomena, while his peers and younger colleagues were branching out into clinical and applied psychology, and resorting to originally banned methods. Thus the advent of behaviorism, Gestalt psychology, mental measurement, and psychoanalysis left structuralism high and dry, and as William McDougall once remarked of Titchener to the present writer, "His psychology proved to be sterile, leading nowhere." That may be an exaggeration; for in his *Elementary Psychology of Feeling and Attention*, and especially in his *Experimental Psychology of the Thought Processes*, there is much sound information of an historical character and not a little wisdom. When he died of a brain tumor in his sixtieth year, Titchener was engaged on a voluminous work on systematic psychology. He was a conscientious and eager translator. Wundt owed much to him in that respect, and his own textbooks enjoyed wide popularity through translations into half a dozen European languages.

MUNSTERBERG
The Pioneer in Applied Psychology

Hugo Münsterberg (1863-1916) was the opposite number of Titchener. They both studied at Leipzig under Wundt, and both were called to America the same year, 1892. Each directed a rival laboratory, among the best in the world. Fundamentally they held the same view as regards systematic psychology, though Titchener was a Wundt stalwart, while Münsterberg broke with Wundt as a young man. Both were introspectionists, Titchener the more rigid of the two. And that is where the resemblances end (except possibly for their hefty physiques).

Münsterberg was teaching at Freiburg im Breisgau, when William James, looking for someone to take over the Harvard Laboratory while he himself was becoming more implicated in the weightier problems of philosophy, came upon Münsterberg's *Die Willenshandlung*. It boldly criticized Wundt's theory that we have an awareness of our will in the sensation of effort, Münsterberg maintaining instead that this sense of effort was due to the message we receive from the muscles, tendons, and joints, and not from the current leaving the brain. Here was a promising ally, James thought; for he, too, disliked Wundt's psychology, and the twenty-nine-year-old Münsterberg somewhat hesitantly accepted the invitation—hesitantly because to him Germany was God's own country, and America a sort of Philistia.

It did not take long for the young psychologist to adapt himself to the needs of the unpromised land;

and he became the foremost promoter of psychology in the country, writing popular books on industrial efficiency, criminology, education, social psychology, business psychology, and the First World War (indicating that his sympathies were with Germany).

Unlike Titchener, Münsterberg never abandoned philosophy. He propounded a double-entry system by which we can appreciate, will, *understand, evaluate* on a *purposive* plane, but *investigate* only according to *causal* standards. He did not, therefore, have the conflicts and problems of James, e.g., in the case of free will *vs.* determinism.

Münsterberg was a first-class experimenter and a director of research par excellence, but, unlike Titchener, he courted glory in various spheres, hobnobbed with royalty and statesmen, made contacts with high-placed persons, and figured in the news. What with serving as an expert in court actions, exposing mediums, advising commissions, he began more and more to neglect the laboratory, leaving it to his assistant, H. S. Langfeld, although he seemed always to be *au courant* with the progress of graduate students, to whom he would assign topics to be investigated for their doctoral dissertations.

In addition to his popular volumes there are several works which made his reputation in the scientific world—*Beiträge zur experimentellen Psychologie, Grundzüge der Psychologie,* and the large work, *Grundzüge der Psychotechnik.* His action theory purported to explain the attributes of sensations as well as the genesis and course of attention, and enjoyed a vogue during his lifetime. Due to overwork and the tension of his involvement during the World War, he died of a cerebral hemorrhage in his fifty-third year, leaving some thirty books, including a small volume of verse. His versatility proved to be a dubious blessing, but there is no doubt that he was one of the giants of American psychology, even if he spurned American citizenship.

LIGHTNER WITMER (1867-1956)— Founder of First Psychological Clinic

Lightner Witmer did not make much of a dent in psychology as such, for he did not bother about systems and was too critical of his more recognized colleagues to have been accepted by the powers that were. But he was a pioneer in that, as professor at the University of Pennsylvania, in 1896, he opened the first psychological clinic, thus paving the way for the hundreds of clinics now in operation. In 1897, he founded the *Psychological Clinic,* a periodical which was continued by his daughter.

Witmer did not take to the rising conceptions of psychiatry and psychoanalysis. He was a realist and wanted to help the child handicapped by deafness or reading deficiency or social maladaptation, through methods which he considered those of common sense. Thus in more influential quarters his labors seemed out of touch with the *Zeitgeist.* His work, however, led to expansion in the fields of vocational guidance, remedial speech and education.

THE ANGRY YOUNG MAN IN PSYCHOLOGY

John Broadus Watson (1878-1958) was not so young when, in 1913, he wrote his *Psychology as the Behaviorist Views It,* thus becoming the spearhead of what was thought to be a new school, labeled "Behaviorism," which behaved like some of the angry young men of our own day.

Was Watson its founder, as is commonly believed? We have seen that the first American behaviorist was James Rush. Before him the French philosopher, Auguste Comte, and his disciple, A. A. Cournot, made the same strictures against introspective psychology as did Watson a century later. Watson proclaimed a new deal for psychology, unaware of the objective psychology of Pavlov and Bekhterev, let alone the less conspicuous work in animal psychology and its anti-introspectionist conclusions by Bethe, Nuel, Beer and von Uexküll.

He took no cognizance of the fact that McDougall, in 1912, had already defined psychology as "the science of behavior." Yet no sooner had Watson's *Behavior; an Introduction to Comparative Psychology* come out, in 1914, than many of the younger instructors began to hail the rebel; and when Watson's publisher, in 1919, sent out complimentary copies of his behavioristic textbook, *Psychology,* it was adopted in a number of colleges as the last word in psychology.

Watson, who was an affable person and could pass for a matinee idol, made a strong appeal to the profession, and by dint of repeated tirades and iconoclastic onslaughts he posed as the mouthpiece of all who were weary of traditional psychology. He was humored by the older men as an "*enfant terrible*," and engaged in absurd debates to show that there is no visual imagery, that consciousness does not exist, that thought is only incipient speech, that the feelings are only sex reactions, that personality is only a compound of habits built upon the basis of fear and sexual attraction, that there are no inborn traits but that fear, anger, and the germ of sex alone are evidenced in the neonate, that he could make any child put in his care in infancy into a genius or a criminal.

Indeed, the number of his unproven assertions mounted as they provoked no serious protest, but, because of his literary connections, were prominently publicized in the press. Readers were given to understand that here came the redeemer of psychology, the man who would solve all problems through slot-machine techniques.

Watson was a good experimentalist, proficient with apparatus and brilliant enough in his own narrow field, but the over-all picture was beyond his ken. He remained an ebullient adolescent in his thinking, but being a born publicist—indeed, Madison Avenue could claim him as its own—he was able to promote the movement until his gross pretensions began to pall in academic circles, and the spread of Gestalt psychology and psychoanalytic doctrines dampened the behavioristic ardor. A moderate behaviorism along the lines of Pavlov's reflexology still rules many laboratories, in the form of operationism, but that is the heritage of mechanism or physicalism

—in short, objectivism, which favors techniques and automatically recorded data. Operationism deserves the niche which it has earned, so long as it does not invade the whole territory, or exclude everything which it cannot handle.

ROBERT S. WOODWORTH

Robert S. Woodworth (1869-) is a distinguished psychologist, genial and amiable, but whether he belongs among the pioneers, founders, discoverers, and theoreticians of a high order, is doubtful. He himself, in his autobiographical sketch, puts it in these words: "I have done comparatively little investigation on my own account. Probably my bent is more toward weighing evidence and 'seeing straight' than toward active enterprise. I should have liked to be a discoverer, so that anyone asking 'What did Woodworth do?' Would be promptly answered, 'Why he is the man who found out this or that.' It is likely that many other psychologists have the same feeling of disillusionment. It seems as if real discoveries, on a par with some in the other sciences, simply were not made in psychology." [8]

For all that; in his long life Woodworth has accomplished a good deal besides teaching mathematics and, later, a dozen different courses in psychology. In the first place, he was an unusually well-trained man, having as teachers, in addition to his "master," J. McKeen Cattell, such celebrities as Charles Sherrington at Liverpool, Külpe at Bonn, Boas and Farrand at Columbia, James and Royce at Harvard, and the physiologists Bowditch and Porter at Harvard and Schafer at Edinburgh. For fellow students, he enjoyed the companionship of E. L. Thorndike and Walter Cannon.

Motivation

Woodworth's contributions began with a monograph on the perception of movement. Of much greater consequence was his collaboration in Ladd's *Elements of Physiological Psychology,* which became the standard work on the subject. His *Dynamic Psychology,* a smallish book, shows him sympathetic to the dynamic school, which is understandable in the light of his early interest in motivation. It was Woodworth who introduced the term "drive" in place of "instinct" in psychology. What makes him a dynamic psychologist is not only the emphasis on drives and motives but his allowance of inference as a method of securing data. Because of the large classes at Columbia, he brought out a textbook which became a best-seller. Written in a colloquial style, it nevertheless had behind it the authority of a top psychologist.

Woodworth's excursion into testing resulted in his devising, with F. L. Wells in 1911, the Association Tests, and the Psychoneurotic Inventory or Personal Data Sheet, which was used during the First World War to eliminate the mentally unfit for military service.

His crowning work is the large volume on experimental psychology which apparently took almost two decades for him and a collaborator, H. Schlosberg, to complete. He was the author of many papers, in all of which his judicial ability is evident. He always weighed both sides of a proposition and always found the means to conciliate extremes, with analogies or through the exigency of scientific integration. He would for example, not be satisfied with studying the minute cells or particles as ultimates.

The whole structure and function of a given organ must have an equal place in the examination. All the events, physiological, psychological and even sociological, of a phenomenon were to him parts of the general framework to be investigated.

HULL (1884-1952)
ALCMAEON AND ERASISTRATUS

Clark L. Hull was born in Akron, Ohio, in a log cabin and raised on a farm, far from educational facilities. Besieged by illness, he did not complete his academic education until he was thirty-four, when he obtained his doctorate in philosophy at the University of Wisconsin, where he stayed on teaching until he left for Yale.

His engineering studies, as in the case of other well-known psychologists, were dropped as soon as he acquired a taste for more theoretical problems, and yet his knack for building things, his motor aptitude, remained with him, and he was able to combine the two sides of his nature to good advantage. Thus he devised an exposure apparatus and a correlation machine and a number of other working tools that served him in good stead in his varied researches in the fields of aptitude testing, hypnosis, suggestibility, and learning. It was in the latter area that he attempted to do something quite novel, viz., to erect a behavior system based on a deductive theory of rate of learning, with postulates, definitions, etc., reminiscent of the Spinozistic method.

The persistence with which Hull carried on his investigation, blending theory with experiment, stimulated many laboratory psychologists to follow his course. It was his purpose to rule out consciousness from consideration; so we may call him a behaviorist —but one of a peculiar cast in that he tried to fit the facts to the theory, which he formulated in precise terms. His wish was to establish laws to apply to conditioning. He introduced such concepts as intervening variables, such as sHr Ds Er, and response variables. The former don't amount to much in the evaluation, but the latter are highly important. The hypothetical constructs were to provide the basis of the system, globally considered.

Hull aimed to be precise and accurate. His goal was to construct a model which could eventually predict behavior—a species of servo-mechanism for psychologists, but he did not figure on the pace of psychology and on the difficulties inherent in such a system, which instead of simplifying the procedure complicates it with parallel conveyors which are yet interdependent. It was Hull's ambition to treat all behavior quantitatively, but the variables are often so many, and their weights so uncertain, that it would hardly do to set up different sets, and arbitrarily assign this or that datum to one or another set of variables.

Hull's faith, enthusiasm, and persistence are to be admired, and some of his students at Yale became leaders in psychology.

Part II

ABNORMAL AND MEDICAL PSYCHOLOGY

PSYCHOPATHOLOGY

It is odd that with the prevalence of mental disorders from time immemorial, the field of psychiatry should have been so late in developing. References to insanity are found in the Bible, in the sacred books of the East, in Greek drama; and the milder psychoneuroses are evident in numerous ancient characters. Indeed, the prophets were not regarded as of sound mind by the ruling families of Israel and Judah.

In his imperishable *Republic,* Plato draws a vivid picture of the hypochondriacs who "are always doctoring and increasing and complicating their disorders and always fancying that they will be cured by any nostrum which anybody advises them to try . . . and the charming thing is that they deem him their worst enemy who tells them the truth, which is simply that unless they give up eating and drinking and wenching and idling, neither drug nor cautery, nor any other remedy, will avail." (*Jowett's translation*)

This appears so modern that it is hard to believe it was written nearly 2,500 years ago, but great is the wonder that even the cave man was treated for mental diseases by a technique which comes close to our lobectomy. True, the sharp stone used for trephining in the stone age is a far cry from the slick scalpel used now in brain surgery; and still further removed from the mid-twentieth century is the prehistoric *mediate* intention of the operation, although their ultimate goal seems to have been the same, namely, to effect a cure, and from the healed scars found on prehistoric skulls, it would appear that the cave surgeons were more skilled than many trained physicians today. Their avowed purpose in making a hole in the brain was for the evil spirits to leave the patient, but the unimagined side effect was to reduce the pressure in the brain by lessening the amount of tissue and fluid. In other words, these cave therapists "builded better than they knew" when they destroyed part of the cerebral substance.

Eastern Practices

As might be anticipated, during the ages of which we have records, religion played an important part in the treatment of mental disorders. Not only under the Sumerian civilization and in ancient Egypt and Assyria, but in Biblical times and in the far Orient, the priests were the physicians too. Sometimes the Hebrew prophets would rebel and demonstratively engage in eccentric behavior, claiming that it was at God's behest, thus rendering themselves open to the charge of being deranged.

Wherever mysticism rules a community, it becomes difficult to establish the demarcation line between the normal and the abnormal. For instance, in India, which has always been steeped in mystic thought, acts which we should consider "crazy" are often in keeping with some particular religious view. The Hindu doctrine of the transmigration of souls, in some measure coinciding with the transformation myths of Greek literature, lends itself to a good deal of superstition, so that a raving madman might be taken for a divine agent. And even today, the cow is protected from the slightest molestation lest the incarnated spirit which may dwell in her be angered.

Plato, in his mystic phase, thought that there were two kinds of madness: the higher lunacy which is peculiar to genius, and the ordinary type. He represented Socrates as receiving his inspiration from the *daimon* that constantly attended him. Here, in the thoughts of a philosopher perhaps without equal, we find the more rational germ of a monstrous demonology which came later.

GRAECO-ROMAN PSYCHIATRY

HIPPOCRATES (*c.* 460-377 B.C.)—
Originator of Temperament Theory

Greek psychiatry, as it may be called by courtesy, or *in embryone,* is centered in the views of the greatest medical mind of antiquity.

Regarded as the father of medicine, Hippocrates was far in advance of his time, and adumbrated some of the modern medical theories. In psychology, his name is associated with the doctrine of the temperaments, which he thought were due to a certain mixture of the humors in the body. He might, therefore, be said to have had an organic approach to mental illness. He described a number of *states* like euphoria and depression, senile dementia and hysteria, which for over 2,400 years was associated solely with the dislodgement of the womb—hence its name (*hysterikos,* Greek for womb).

Hippocrates' aperçus at times foreshadowed the findings of today. He noted, for example, the apparent superinduction of one pathological condition through another which, although bad in itself, may be relatively better than the original disease, on the principle that we ought to choose the lesser of two evils. The intuitive grasp of Hippocrates, who was what might today be called a phenomenalist rather than an inductive experimentalist, appears in his examination of patients along the lines of individual differences, so that each one might be handled separately rather than by rule of thumb.

He was a practical physician who applied his results in a professional manner instead of spinning out theories based on speculation. He could see the excesses of some of his colleagues in bleeding an unfortunate to death or purging the sick to utter exhaustion. Prudence and moderation were the basis of his highly reputed and affluent practice. He evinced little interest in the oracles and superstitions of the day; and thus, no matter how inadequate his knowledge of physiology, he clung steadfastly to the frame of reference which constituted his calling.

There were other physicians in Greece worthy of our admiration. Alcmaeon, perhaps the first to do dissecting (of animals), lived in the latter part of the sixth century B.C. and was referred to occasionally by Aristotle. Herophilus and Erasistratus were contemporaries of Theophrastus, Aristotle's successor as head of the Peripatetic School. Herophilus, scion of the Asclepiades family, was the originator of the autopsy, and through his dissection of the brain, made a number of discoveries in anatomy. The duodenum was so named because he found that this intestine was about twelve finger breadths long. He had little truck with the prevailing doctrine of the humors, in the etiology of the day, and attributed aberrations to a defective nervous system, which he located in the brain. Of his writings only a tract on respiration is preserved in manuscript.

Erasistratus, the son of Aristotle's daughter, was so devoted to anatomical research that he gave up his practice. Certain parts of the brain and the auricles of the heart were first described in detail by him. Like his friend, Herophilus, he had no use for bloodletting or purgation, and prescribed instead warm baths, dieting, exercise, and if necessary emetics. More important for our purpose was his discernment of allergies, which, following a lead of Hippocrates, he subsumed under the term "idiosyncrasy." Erasistratus believed the vital impulse converged, as air, through the arteries, while the veins were sufficient to carry the blood, essential for vitalizing the system, both producing and sustaining the warmth of the body.

Around 150 B.C., the great medical center at Alexandria, because of squabbles and rivalries, was soon transferred to Rome. Among the men who adumbrated modern psychopathology, Asclepiades ranks high. He made many distinctions, such as acute and chronic disease, fevers as against mental ills, delusions and hallucinations, the more agitated and milder derangements; and was the first to treat the mentally ill by psychotherapy, devising means of making them more relaxed and physically comfortable.

Cicero is so completely associated with rhetoric and statesmanship that to many it may come as a surprise to learn that he was also preoccupied with "diseases of the soul," as he called them. Both he and Plutarch, who describes what we popularly call the "nervous breakdown," with its self-accusation, listlessness, exhaustion, and guilt feelings, must have given thought to the subject. Another literary man who compiled a sort of medical encyclopedia or handbook, *De Re Medica*—incidentally, the first medical work in Latin—was Celsus. However, not being a physician, his attitude differed from the humane approach of Asclepiades, for instance. He advocated a rigid regimen to shock patients into coming to their senses, recommending punishment for violations as well as the ordinary physical nostrums, which the trained practitioners were beginning to discard.

ARETAEUS

A man who had an impact on later minds, even the celebrated Galen a century later, was Aretaeus, who came from Cappadocia and flourished about 80 A.D. His earlier interests were in what we call organic medicine—indigestion, ulcers in the throat, jaundice, and paralysis, which he attributed to intestinal disorders. The abdomen also received much of his attention, figuring together with the head as the locus of mental ills. Aretaeus was the first to recognize that mania and depression are but two phases of the same disease, and he associated one phase with youth and the other with advanced age, looking for the causes in the different blood temperatures. The clinical pictures which Aretaeus draws are remarkable for his time, and his observations sound modern in some respects. According to Zilboorg, "Aretaeus was the first known to become interested, interested as we are today, in the personalities of the people who later develop severe mental diseases." It may be said that he paved the way for Jung and Kretschmer. Another of his specialties was the art of prognosis, which, except for the eminent Archigenes, was practically unknown at the time. He seems to have been a down-to-earth seeker of the simple explanation. He did not believe in the divine source of the creative inspiration sometimes exhibited by the insane, ascribing it rather to their background.

SORANUS OF EPHESUS

Two genuine pioneers of methods in handling the insane were Soranus and Caelius Aurelianus, who translated Soranus into Latin before the original manuscript was lost. From Soranus' vivid accounts of various patients, we can see that so far as delusions are concerned, they have not changed in two thousand years.

Soranus rails at the intellectualistic approach to therapy. Some of his predecessors did not take into consideration that the sufferer fails to reason, and that penalties or hardships would not be conducive to improvement. Soranus was the harbinger of humane treatment, even though his voice did not carry into the new era of darkness. The hit-or-miss recipes of his peers and colleagues were exposed with irresistible logic as calculated to worsen a condition rather than cure it. Homeopathic medicine was not dreamed of, and Soranus was constantly trying to avoid ill consequences, even to the extent of interdicting sexual intercourse in many instances, since he was not sure whether the state of depression consequent upon the act, according to the saying "*post coitus omne animal triste*" was not more detrimental than the restlessness due to the restriction.

CAELIUS AURELIANUS

Of the same stripe as Soranus was Caelius Aurelianus, a North African, most likely of Semitic stock, which might explain in part his abhorrence of Graeco-Roman sex practices, growing worse during the second century in Rome. His primary service to organic medicine was his study of hydrophobia, which he considered an affliction centered largely in the splanchnic nerves.

From Aurelianus, who was affiliated with the so-called methodist school in ancient medicine, we obtain a pretty full survey of medical doings in the first two centuries of the Christian era. In his *De Morbis Acutis et Chronicis,* he delivers a few significant observations in regard to treatment, which contravened the practices of the day, such as deploring the castration of epileptics as a form of therapy. He made an inventory of symptoms according to the types of dementia, and cautioned against diagnosing from one or two symptoms.

In other words, he already understood the need of a concept like "syndrome," without actually formulating it. Nor did he exclude the conclusions of other physicians than those belonging to his school. Whether from his own practice or his vast readings, he manipulated deftly a wealth of facts, largely of a symptomatic nature, and proved himself an extraordinarily judicious sifter. The influence of the speculative philosophers he deemed bad, confining his attention to observable data and allowing for a certain amount of extrapolation.

THE GREAT GALEN (*c.* 131-205)—
Formulator of the Humors Doctrine

We come now to the colossus of ancient medicine, the most influential medical writer after Hippocrates, whom he follows and elaborates—the great Claudius Galenus, or simply Galen, as he is known to the moderns, who served as a beacon casting its beams down the centuries of medieval dusk, through the Renaissance, and up to the Enlightenment period.

Born in 131, in Pergamus, Asia Minor, from which we derive the word "parchment," he received a good education, especially in medicine, and was soon off to Alexandria, the Mecca of prospective physicians. At the age of thirty-four, we find him in Rome, where he was already known for his learning and skill, becoming the archiater of no less a philosopher-emperor than Marcus Aurelius. His efforts to train physicians in the intricacies of anatomy were cut short by jealousies and animosities that did not tend to soften his congenitally impulsive nature.

Galen was a scientist who, for all his eclecticism, made important anatomical discoveries, and may be looked upon as the Vesalius of antiquity, despite the errors pointed out more than a thousand years later by the father of modern anatomy. The number of his works, especially when it is considered that he engaged in research as well as in practice, is staggering. Through actual experiments, he proved that the seat of the mind was not the heart, as Aristotle thought, but the brain. He likewise rejected the doctrine of

Erasistratus, that the function of the arteries was to provide air to the body, assigning this function to the windpipe and lungs, while connecting the arteries with the heart, and both with the flow of blood. He missed the discovery of circulation because of his preoccupation with the humoral theory of the temperaments conceived by Hippocrates, which he elaborated so plausibly that for many centuries it remained the all-in-all of medical etiology.

Instead of the original two temperaments, Galen drew up nine, combinations of warm, cold, humid, and dry. Galen distinguished between the choleric and the melancholic temperament, which hitherto had been lumped together under the bilious.

It would seem that Galen's theoretical mind, wishing to correlate facts and seeking causal connections along lines already begun, was diverted from finding the true relationship of organ and function, though it was so close at hand. Yet he left nuggets of wisdom and medical intuitions which must astound us. He rather than Aretaeus, established the recently accepted fact that the proximity of a symptom to a given organ does not necessarily mean that the trouble lies therein.

In his psychological thinking, he might be classed as a realist or perhaps a modern positivist. He believed the soul's functioning depended on the nature of the brain tissue, its coarseness, fineness, heaviness, lightness, and mobility. When he states that mobility is responsible for changes of opinion, he is on territory close to Hobbes, who attributed all thought to the motion of the brain particles.

Throughout his life Galen was in quest of causes and purposes. He assumed that the body was constructed so that each minute part had its why and wherefore; therefore he could not rest satisfied until he had discovered, as he thought, the rationale of its being, as well as its *modus operandi.* In his pursuit of systematization, he emulated Aristotle. To him most of his colleagues were narrow professionals or merely empirics, and in polemic passages throughout his treatise, his disparagement of them sounds almost like superciliousness, born of conceit.

SCIENTIFIC DEBACLE

The death of Galen in 200 A.D. marked the close of the classical period and coincides with the beginning of Roman disintegration, under the degenerate Commodus. His successors made it their business to crush all science. Even the redoubtable Diocletian, an able ruler, was instrumental in the slaughter of many scholars in Alexandria; and with the establishment of Christianity as the state religion, by Constantine in 313, the study of Plato and Aristotle was banned. As Christianity spread and its organization became intrenched and consolidated, the priests and monks, who ministered to their flock and were often the only literate people in a community, took over the function of caring for the sick, especially the mentally ill. Because of its very abnormality, madness was now associated with the supernatural. It was the work of the evil one, the result of commerce between the madman and demons, who were constantly tempting man to perdition.

During an impending cataclysm an eruption of mysticism is natural, in this instance enhanced by the zeal of Christian fanatics. Superstition always rides on the crest of ignorance. The restraining power of classical thought was gone, and a compound of bigotry and obscurantism was about to pay off in atrocities which are blood-curdling to read about.

Alexandria fell to the Arabs in 640, and the last two medical writers to preserve some semblance of a tradition were Alexander of Tralles and Paul of Aegina (in the next century), who was Byzantine in spirit. Alexander, although an inventor of all sorts of concoctions, in which the ingredients often included excrement or blood, was at least conversant with the chief writings of the Greek medical men. Paul was more of a practitioner, who wrote out prescriptions and believed that short cuts, digests, and summaries of the masters were all that was necessary for physicians to acquire. Research became a thing of the past, and practitioners were content with a limited amount of skill, e.g., in child delivery or in lancing. Medical progress came to a dead halt.

THE RISE OF ARABIC MEDICINE

While the scientific sun was setting in the West, the moon, in the form of a crescent, was rising in the East. Certainly its light could not compare with the refulgent brilliance which was the glory of the Alexandrian school in centuries past, but its reflection alone was enough to light the way at a time when Europe was enveloped in darkness, with theology throttling every attempted scientific break-through.

The Western monasteries did house a large number of manuscripts, but little attention was paid to them by the monks and clergy in general, who were for the most part scarcely educated and certainly ignorant of Greek. Happily, the Abbasside Caliphs, who ruled in the Near East during the eighth and ninth centuries, were patrons of the arts and liberal in thought. They brought together a small library of manuscripts and enlisted a translation force of highly competent Syrian, Jewish, Persian, and Greek medical practitioners to translate the most important works of the masters in medicine. Thus started the efflorescence of Arabic medicine, cultivated by Moslems, Jews and Byzantines; and the Baghdad School in what is now Iraq became almost as much of a medical center as Alexandria in the first two centuries, and at least as noted as the Salerno School in the tenth century.

Schools, libraries and hospitals were set up in Mesopotamia, North Africa, and Spain and a literature was created which was characterized more by erudite scholarship than by new discoveries. Avicenna, Rhazes, Haly Abbas, Maimonides, and Albucasis are some of the outstanding men whose works display the Greek influence to a marked degree.[9]

During the Dark Ages, the West had some shining lights, but they moved in a theological sphere. Should anyone veer an iota from accepted dogma, expulsion, as in the case of Nestorius, was the mildest penalty. Burning at the stake was more likely; and Abelard, the greatest mind of his century, barely escaped it.

Great Arab Physicians

Under Moslem rule, religious practice was required, but Nestorius, who fled to Persia, and the Jews, were permitted to continue their labors unmolested. Instead of theology, philosophers of high caliber—such as Averroës (Ibn Roshd), the foremost of the Arab commentators on Aristotle, Avicenna (Ibn Sina) and Maimonides, chose medicine for their profession.

Maimonides, court physician to the celebrated Saladin and his son, did not neglect theology; and he too had bitter opponents among the ultra-orthodox. But he did not have to appear before ecclesiastical bodies, and for all the criticism, he was revered by his brethren throughout the world, while his credo of thirteen principles is repeated daily by millions of Jews today.

His medical writings are based on Hippocrates and Galen, but his manual of hygiene, both physical and mental, contains elaborations of his own, around a core of common sense and personal dignity. His *Hygiene of the Soul* contains detailed descriptions of the depressed, together with advice to the attending physician. He preaches prudence, moderation, and equanimity as vouchsafing good health; and what in present popular circles goes under the name of "positive thinking" is definitely to be found in that *vade mecum* for physicians and the intellectual layman. The style is that of Spinoza's *Improvement of the Understanding*—a personal approach.

West Discovers West Through East

Translation of Greek manuscripts proceeded in a curiously circuitous manner. They were done first into Syriac, which is a later form of Aramaic, and then into Arabic, which is akin to Syriac. The next step was to translate them into Latin. Were it not for Arab and, mainly, Jewish translators, many of these manuscripts would have been lost before the Western world discovered them during the Middle Ages. Scholars with a thorough knowledge of Greek were few and far between. There were exceptions, like Gerard of Cremona, who mastered Arabic so that he could translate the Arabic translations, but it can be imagined how divergent from the original texts the roundabout versions must have been—like the allegory of Plato's shadows in the cave.

DEMONISM

The spurning of the classics was not the worst transgression of Europe during the Dark Ages. As superstition spread among all classes, and Church dogma ruled with an iron hand, abnormal behavior was no longer associated with medicine, but rather with the supernatural and, therefore, was seen as coming under the jurisdiction of theology. Indeed, even ordinary disabilities were related to religion. It was not the physician but God who effects the cure, through the intercession of Mary or the saints. The saints must be appealed to. Prayers and penance became the medicaments, and the clergy took over the function of physician, administering drugs which had religious or astrological implications.

Actually, the treatment possessed all the earmarks of magic. The more ingeniously fantastic the conception, the greater the efficacy ascribed to it. A typical prescription would run as follows: Take a testicle of a goat that has been killed on a Tuesday midnight, during the first quarter of the moon, and the heart of a dog, mix with the excrement of a newborn babe, and after pulverizing, take an amount equivalent to half an olive twice a day. This "dung pharmacopoeia." as it has been dubbed in our enlightened age, enjoyed a vogue even in the American Colonial period. That, along with incantations, or magical formulae, was the order of the day.

Is it so strange, then, that mental ailments should have been traced to dark forces dwelling in hell but roaming invisibly among humans in order to enthrall them and cause their ruination? To be in league with the Devil was the worst crime imaginable; and, according to the Old Testament, no sorcerer or witch should be allowed to live.

The campaign against such wizardry assumed gigantic proportions, and during the sixteenth and seventeenth centuries, hundreds of thousands of the "possessed" were burned, or, as in our own village of Salem, hanged with the approval of intellectual leaders such as Cotton Mather, who had been elected a fellow of the Royal Society in England, and who was not unfamiliar with the best medical treatises of the day.

What could be more natural than to trace every disorder, every catastrophe—and epidemics, droughts, floods, and earthquakes there were aplenty—to unholy connections with the Evil One; and who should be the culprit but the hysteric or manic individual, whose very deviant conduct singled him out as inhuman?

In the knowledge, however, that the Devil would play cozy, the new type physicians developed a new system of diagnosis to ferret out the possessed. Certain moles or *naevi,* a particular kind of squint (evil eye) or cross-eyedness, hyperesthesia or anesthesia, or failing to bleed when pricked, was a sure sign that a person was possessed. A testing apparatus was devised by which anyone could be pricked by agents of the inquisitors; and such symptoms as would have not otherwise have been uncovered were regarded as establishing guilt.

Friars and abbots, bishops, and even popes became uneasy about the possible consequences of a growing demonic onslaught. To make matters worse, hysterics, largely women, would confess heinous sins, and act as if they were really possessed. The only cure was burning, generally preceded by torture. The erotic aspect of hysteria appeared in the women's stories of sexual intercourse with the "Fiend."

That women were the victims for the most part is due partly to their suggestibility, emotionality, and greater susceptibility to hysteria than men; but we must also bear in mind that they were the scapegoats, who received the blame for anything that went wrong. It is estimated that for every man convicted as a sorcerer, there were fifty "witches," and that at least 150,000 of them were executed, most of them after abusive treatment, such as being brought to trial naked, with all hair shaved, but not facing the judges, lest they bewitch them; and in some cases bruised or maimed.

The "Hammer"

When the populace in some of the more enlightened places did not take kindly to such high-handed methods and questionable techniques of probing, two Dominican monks, Heinrich Kraemer and Johann Sprenger, took it upon themselves to convince the world. Their lucubration, citing chapter and verse became the Bible of all witch-hunters, and its authors, toward the end of 1484, received the approval of Pope Innocent VIII, to act as inquisitors in the task of eradicating the evil. This infamous compendium, called *Malleus Maleficarum* (*Hammer of the Witches*), with its euphonious assonance, was, indeed, more than a hammer. It was an instrument of mass murder. The Dominican "dogs of the Lord" (*canes Domini*), as they styled themselves, were wolves on the prowl, serpents insidiously pouncing on their prey; and the deadly effect of their poisonous fangs penetrated all Christendom, even to far-off New England, with its Calvinist setting.

It was not long before the behavior of ordinary people began to be scrutinized by their neighbors and reported as bearing out the symptomatology of the handbook. As in the case of authoritarian governments in our own time, to be accused sealed the fate of the suspect. Those who nursed grievances found an easy way to square themselves with their enemies. International chicanery discovered a new device for dealing with delicate problems. Joan of Arc, the "Maid of Orleans," who, at the age of seventeen, dauntlessly led the French army to victory, was later betrayed and burned as a witch. To the ecclesiastical judges her hallucinations meant only one thing, that she was in communication with the Devil. That she was later canonized by the Church whose representatives had her burned hardly mitigates the grievousness of the crime.

The *Hammer* appeared only a few years before the discovery of America. The Dominicans, the most powerful and obscurantist order of the Church, were about to come to grips with a new force—the Reformation. They moved heaven and earth to crush every semblance of enlightenment. Every book which ran counter to their special dogmas, no matter how ancient, was ordered consigned to the flames. With the help of a former Jewish butcher, an outcast by the name of Pfefferkorn, an ignoramus posing as a rabbi, they engineered a scheme to have the Talmud burned. Their political artifices almost proved successful, but for the learning and courage of the great Johann Reuchlin, Nestor of the Humanists, and harbinger of the Reformation, and his coadjutors, who produced the most remarkable satire of all times—the *Epistolae Virorum Obscurorum,* parodies of letters supposedly written by Dominicans, which exposed their inferior Latin style and incorrect grammar, as well as their intrigues and lasciviousness.

The witch-hunters were soon to encounter mighty spirits like Erasmus, Melanchthon, Sir Thomas More, and the most militant of all, Martin Luther, whose nailing of the ninety-five theses on a Wittenberg church door, in 1517, was the *défi* which heralded the Reformation. Curiously enough, Luther himself was said to have thrown inkwells at the Devil, whom he hallucinated, and was not much more tolerant than those he fought.

The martyrdom of countless innocent victims was not restricted to any single region or country. Witch-hunting became a favorite pastime, affording an outlet for the hostility and aggression common to mankind, especially since it was rationalized as a sacred duty. Of viciousness born of bigotry—or perhaps the sequence should be reversed—the Dominicans had no monopoly. In the British Colonies, which constituted a refuge for the Puritans who fled from religious restriction, the same tendency manifested itself, without benefit of official inquisitors.

Hangings of Hysterical Women

One could hardly have wished for a more intelligent community than the one in Salem, close to Boston, toward the end of the seventeenth century, more than two hundred years after the appearance of the *Malleus Maleficarum*. Yet in 1692, in little Salem alone, nineteen respectable women were hanged as witches and Giles Corey, who apparently defied the magistrates at the trial, was pressed to death. Chief witnesses against the unfortunates were a few hysterical teen-agers. If the antics of rock-'n-rollers had occurred during those days, they would doubtless have been seen as manifestations of sorcery, incited by the Prince of Darkness.

E. W. Taylor, writing on the subject, summarizes the condition as bearing "the stamp of 'group hysteria' in which suggestion, self-protection, a feeling of domination, in an atmosphere of profound belief in the activity of witchcraft, played a predominant role. The spirit of mischief and maliciousness was certainly subordinate." [10]

One might suppose that these executions, or legal murders, would be denounced by every intelligent person in our century, but Barrett Wendell, a noted Harvard English professor, thought that the condemned were not actually guileless, for in his opinion, they indulged in all sorts of psychic phenomena, trances, mediumships, etc., and therefore laid themselves open to serious charges. His more distinguished colleague, E. L. Kittredge, pleads extenuating circumstances on behalf of Judge Sewall and his associates, as well as Cotton Mather, who favored the executions. It is even alleged that the latter, arguing privately against the defense, approved the verdict as the "will of the Lord."

MODERN DEMONISM

More astounding is the fact that a belief in demonism is by no means dead in our own civilization; and I am not thinking of the "hex" stories involving murders we sometimes read about in the newspapers. Some of those who take stock in the existence of demons whose business is to torment humans are highly educated. There is for instance, Rev. Hugh W. White, a Presbyterian missionary and doctor of divinity, who is familiar with the psychopathology of Charcot, Janet, Freud, Jung, Adler, A. Meyer, Sidis, Morton Prince, and other therapists, and yet, in 1922, published a book entitled *Demonism Verified and Analyzed,* in which he employs scientific terminology, and cites the psychological literature, to build up his thesis on the basis of cases which he claims to have dealt with personally.

Chapter 7, "Satanic Origin of Demonism," opens with the statement: "In all ages, men have tried to disprove or laugh off the fact that the world has an enemy, Satan, who works against all that is good. The facts of demonism confirm the Bible on this point." He holds that: (a) demonism cannot be classed with the other insanities; (b) it cannot be accounted for on merely pathological grounds; and (3) it allows for the demonizing of the healthy as well as of the pathological.

There is some close reasoning in the book, but let us quote a passage which will afford an insight into the minds of the judges who consigned hysterical women to the flames or the scaffold.

> On February 13, 1921, we began a Bible class at the village Tienhu, to meet every day for a week. On that day, Sunday, after the meeting, a woman, my No. 435, came forward holding a baby. She looked normal and happy. I had not noticed her in the congregation. She said she had been demonized, but was healed, and she wanted us to pray for the baby. While we are praying all of a sudden the woman herself breaks out shouting as the demon saying, "Not vex little one, vex big one." The face is now vicious-looking, underlip sucked in, eyes lowering. She turns slowly round and round. I order the demon to leave her. The reply is, "I have nowhere to go." I order the demon to kneel to Jesus. The reply is, "I will not kneel." But, in a minute or two, I notice a weakening of the patient's aspect, and make her lie down. There is a slight eructation. I tell the people the demon is gone. Presently she goes out with a Christian woman, normal.[11]

When we consider the state of the human mind during the Dark Ages, with its welter of beliefs and theories, alchemical, astrological, and cabbalistic—all drenched in superstition—we can understand how the *Malleus* of the two Dominicans could have passed through no less than thirty editions between 1487 and 1669, at a time when reading was an accomplishment of the few.

But why waste our wonderment on those who lived centuries back; when we have before us the Introduction, written by Montague Summers, *anno* 1946, to the English translation by John Rodker, in which Summers declares that "It is not too much to say that the *Malleus Maleficarum* is among the most important, wisest, and weightiest books of the world."

That it is an amazing disquisition there can be no doubt. Sprenger and Kraemer were learned in their own way, quoting from Aristotle as well as the Church authorities, and arguing methodically in Teutonic and Scholastic fashion. The stories they accumulated afford us a picturesque view of the medieval mind, and particularly pinpoint the ideas of the masses. The work is a treasury of folklore; and is correctly so catalogued in large secular university libraries as the one at Harvard University.

SEX PRACTICES OF THE "DEVIL"

Some of the problems which the authors discuss are truly entrancing. Raising questions about sexual relations between witches and devils—which, of course, they take for granted—they purport to answer them in the manner of scientists discussing, say, phenomena in physics or chemistry.

Here follows the Way whereby Witches copulate with those Devils known as Incubi.

> As to the method in which witches copulate with Incubus devils, six points are to be noted. First, as to the devil and the body which he assumes, of what element it is formed. Second, as to the act, whether it is always accompanied with the injection of semen, received from some other man. Third, as to the time and place, whether one time is more favorable than another for this practice. Fourth, whether the act is visible to the women, and whether only those who were begotten in this way are so visited by devils. Fifth, whether it applies only to those who were offered to the devil at birth by midwives. Sixth, whether the actual venereal pleasure is greater or less in this act.[12]

ARTIFICIAL INSEMINATION

Basing some of their conclusions on the authority of St. Thomas, who apparently believed that "those begotten in this way by devils are more powerful than other men," they come close to the conception of artificial, or at least indirect, insemination. When the question of the injection of semen is taken up, we are told that no infallible rule can be advanced. It all depends. If the witch is old and sterile, then the devil will not waste his substance, as he is seeking results; and an efficient agent must be productive, to use modern business terms.

> But if she is not sterile, he approaches her in the way of carnal delectation which is procured for the witch. And should she be disposed to pregnancy, then if he can conveniently possess the semen extracted from some man, he does not delay to approach her with it, for the sake of infecting her progeny.
>
> But if it is asked whether he is able to collect the semen emitted in some nocturnal pollution in sleep, just as he collects that which is spent in the carnal act, the answer is that it is probable that he cannot, though others hold a contrary opinion. For it must be noted that, as has been said, the devils pay attention to the generative virtue which is more abundant and better preserved in semen obtained by the carnal act, being wasted in the semen that is due to nocturnal pol-

lutions in sleep, which arises from the superfluity of the humours and is not emitted with great generative virtue.[13]

Another problem to be solved by the authors is whether the devil is visible in the midst of his orgy; and with a show of common sense they argue that he certainly is visible to the witch who is in pact with him.

> But with regard to any bystanders, the witches themselves have often been seen lying on their backs in the fields or the woods naked up to the very navel, and it has been apparent from the disposition of those limbs and members which pertain to the venereal act and orgasm, as also from the agitation of their legs and thighs, that, all invisibly to the bystanders, they have been copulating with Incubus devils; yet sometimes howbeit this is rare, at the end of the act a very black vapour, of about the stature of a man, rises up into the air from the witch.[14]

SEXUAL PRANKS OF THE "DEVIL"

The authors are

> certain also that the following has happened. Husbands have actually seen Incubus devils swiving their wives, although they have thought that they were not devils but men. And when they have taken up a weapon and tried to run them through, the devil has suddenly disappeared, making himself invisible. And then their wives have thrown their arms about them, although they have sometimes been hurt, and railed at their husbands, mocking them, and asking them if they had eyes, or whether they were possessed of the devils.[15]

Naturally, it occurred to the authors that impotence is often caused by the devils. Everything is set before us explicitly, in Part II:

> Intrinsically they cause it in two ways. First, when they directly prevent the erection of the member which is accommodated to fructification. And this need not seem impossible, when it is considered that they are able to vitiate the natural use of any member. Secondly, when they prevent the flow of the vital essences to the members in which resides the motive force, closing up the seminal ducts so that it does not reach the generative vessels, or so that it cannot be ejaculated, or is fruitlessly spilled.

Extrinsically they cause it at times by means of images, or by the eating of herbs; sometimes by other external means, such as cocks' testicles. But it must not be thought that it is by the virtue of these things that a man is made impotent; but by the occult power of devils' illusions. Witches by this means procure such impotence, namely, that they cause a man to be unable to copulate, or a woman to conceive.[16]

On the strength of their reports, it is to be understood that by some trick of the devil, a man may find himself despoiled of his genitals. In this book of wisdom we are treated to the following delectable morsel:

"And what, then, is to be thought of those witches who in this way sometimes collect male organs in great numbers, as many as twenty or thirty members together, and put them in a bird's nest, or shut them up in a box, where they move themselves like living members, and eat oats and corn, as has been seen by many and is a matter of common report? It is to be said that it is all done by devil's work and illusion, for the senses of those who see them are deluded in the way we have said. For a certain man tells that, when he had lost his member, he approached a known witch to ask her to restore it to him. She told the afflicted man to climb a certain tree, and that he might take which he liked out of a nest in which there were several members. And when he tried to take a big one, the witch said: "You must not take that one"; adding, "because it belonged to a parish priest."[17]

RULES FOR TORTURE

The third part of the *Malleus* is the most useful from our point of view. since here is sketched the course of procedure in apprehending, trying, convicting, and executing the witches. Evidently it was written by the co-author, who was an authority on jurisprudence. It is a scholarly treatise taking up issues step by step, and dealing with every point in detail: the fitness of the judges, examination of witnesses, type of questioning, eliciting confession, method of sentencing, etc. The author uses the case of the Jew in canonical law as an analogy or precedent for the treatment of witches. "Besides in the last canon law concerning Jews it says: 'His goods are to be confiscated, and he is to be condemned to death, because with perverse doctrine he opposed the Faith of Christ.'" Why then should we be surprised at the following set of instructions, which were apparently adopted by all magistrates who came under the jurisdiction of Pope Innocent VIII?

> And while she is being questioned about each several point, let her be often and frequently exposed to torture beginning with the more gentle of them; for the Judge should not be too hasty to proceed to the graver kind. And while this is being done, let the Notary write all down, how she is tortured and what questions are asked and how she answers.

> And note that, if she confesses under torture, she should then be taken to another place and questioned anew so that she does not confess only under the stress of torture.[18]

> The next step of the Judge should be that, if after being fittingly tortured, she refuses to confess the truth, he should have other engines of torture brought before her, and tell her that she will have to endure these if she does not confess. If then she is not induced by terror to confess, the torture must be continued on the second or third day, but not repeated at that present time unless there should be some fresh indication of its probable success.

It is said Kraemer and Sprenger were pious and energetic men. Without a doubt they were zealous and efficient, but after all allowance is made for the period, their perverseness, uncritical judgment, and sheer cruelty remain unforgivable. Hundreds of thousands of innocent men and women were tortured to death as a result of their—considering their designation, *canes Domini*—doggedness.

That enlightened men lived during those centuries goes without saying, but few of them had the courage to counter the authority of the Inquisitors or the finality of a Papal Bull. Men like Giordano Bruno, Rabelais, John of Salisbury, Roger Bacon, Thomas More, Ambroise Paré, or Michel Montaigne were rare; and nearly all of them paid the price of nonconformity, if not the extreme penalty, at least imprisonment, abuse, and humiliation.

CORNELIUS AGRIPPA—Spiritual Warrior

In the stronghold of the fanatical Dominicans—Cologne—in 1486, at about the time the *Witches' Hammer* began to pound innocent women, a child was born into the world feet first, and, according to the custom of the time, was called Agrippa, a sort of portmanteau name, derived from *aegritudo* (to suffer pain) and *pes* (foot). Apparently, Agrippa was conscious of his name and expressed its meaning in his own crusading propensities.

Endowed in many ways, he took doctorates in theology, law, and medicine, and was therefore fully acquainted with the misdeeds of the three most important professions. But he was also valiant on the battlefield, and invented an early version of the telescope as well as a death weapon. His life should have been well filled and well contented, but paradoxically, most of it was a veritable nightmare; and the denigration of his character, on the part of his enemies, was so complete that even after his death, his name became associated in the world at large with the vilest deeds, while his black French poodle was identified with the Devil.

Even such a free spirit as Rabelais could not forget that Agrippa had written a book on occult philosophy wherein he showed that, through a process of counting and applying certain astrological symbols, one could foretell what would happen in certain houses. In his great satire (Chapter XXV), Rabelais refers to Agrippa's ("Her Trippa," he calls him) proficiency in all the "mancies," like geomancy, chiromancy, necromancy, etc. He knows what is happening in every house, yet does not suspect that his own third wife is cuckolding him, while he assures Panurge, who consults him, that if he marries, all the signs in every divine art point to his ending up a cuckold. It is a pitiless lampoon, all the more so since Agrippa had died a short time before.

Rabelais took no note of Agrippa's gifts and learning, his abandonment of the occult hodgepodge, and his critical pronouncements on science and the arts (*De incertitudine et vanitate scientarum et artum*). If Agrippa had been instrumental in saving only a single woman from the clutches of the Inquisition, he would deserve our gratitude, but he actually jeopardized his life by denouncing its tortures and executions.

He might have accomplished much in medical research, had he been settled and secure, but restlessness and rebelliousness played havoc with his potentialities. He was continually harassed and hounded by his enemies; and he had a special knack for multiplying them with his sharp tongue and trenchant pen.

Since his earlier interests were of the esoteric kind, and Cabbala with its promise of achieving miracles through the correct formulation of the tetragrammaton (IHWH) had been the desideratum of the learned since the days of Pico della Mirandola, Agrippa studied and subsequently taught Hebrew at Dôle, using Reuchlin's little book on the "wonder-working word." We next find him in England, in Italy, and then in Maximilian's army where he distinguished himself and was created a knight. In Metz, he became city attorney and saved a woman from burning at the stake as a witch, but that great crime was enough to incite the powerful fanatics and those citizens who had been cheated of a thrill. Agrippa was fortunate enough to escape in time. In his fight to release the girl, who was subject to torture so that she might confess her intercourse with the Devil, because her mother had been burned as a witch, he called the fat Dominican Inquisitor, Nicolas Savin, a hypocrite who hid his iniquity under the cover of the Gospel. It was in the same city that Inquisitor Savin had had an opponent, Jean Le Clerk, tortured, flogged publicly as a steady diet, and then given orders to cut off his nose and right hand, and after causing hot metal to be placed on his head, finished up the job by having him consigned to the flames. That, in the name of religion, in the name of Jesus!

For a few years Agrippa enjoyed comparative peace in Friburg, Switzerland, where he practiced medicine; but his venturesome spirit soon drove him to France, where, at Lyons, he became the physician-astrologer to Louise, mother of François I. He was dismissed when he would not reveal her horoscope, possibly because it bode no good. In 1528, he went to the Netherlands and was imprisoned for over a year. He then turned up in his birthplace, Cologne, where he was engaged as the Emperor's historiographer, but again the Dominicans, intrenched in their own capital, made life miserable for him, and he was forced to take refuge in Grenoble, France, where he died shortly thereafter, in 1535.

Thus was cut short, at the age of forty-nine, the life of an intellectual warrior who influenced his younger contemporary, Paracelsus, through his ideas on magnetism and the relationship between the microcosm and the macrocosm. He exerted more direct impact upon a youth who was to become the "Hammer" of the *Witches' Hammer* and its votaries. In a sense, he removed the brambles from the path to the inwardly disturbed, and thus opened the road for the development of psychiatry. Johann Weyer must have been spurred by the tribulations which Agrippa, his first teacher, had to endure as a result of the obscurantism of the age and the sadism of its executive officers.

It may be true, as R. M. Lawrence says that Agrippa was "an earnest searcher after truth who was fain to attempt the unlocking of nature's secrets but did not hold the right key." Certainly his mind leaned too much toward the irrational, as, for example, when he thought that the manner in which an herb was cut had to do with its efficacy as a cure, but it cannot be denied that he was a meteor lighting up the dark sky of a particularly dismal period.

PARACELSUS, Mystic and Scientist

As we approach the peak of the Renaissance and the Reformation, we see the birth of more and more enlightened spirits—among them Paracelsus (1493-1541). Paracelsus would have been an extraordinary character in any age, but at the dawn of humanism, he looms as a strange blend of mysticism and practicalness. We are reminded of another great mystic whose technical efficiency, two centuries later, made him the favorite of king and emperor. That was Swedenborg, who before the illumination which he experienced at the age of fifty-four, was a mining and financial wizard, counselor of the mighty, and the author of technological works, and thereafter began to explore the heavens and hell, to communicate with angels, and eventually to found a new cult.

The mysticism of Paracelsus was in keeping with his time. He believed in astrology, in lunar influences, in some of the medical claptrap which had been afloat since the days of Galen. But at the same time he was an iconoclast, and it mattered little to him who the idol was that he was about to smash.

His very name tells a story. His actual name was Theophrastus Bombastus von Hohenheim. His eponym, Theophrastus (meaning "god-counseled") was Aristotle's successor in Athens, a sage in the best sense and the father of literary characterology. The rest of his name, Bombastus von Hohenheim, does sound a bit pompous even for a sprig of the nobility, and he can hardly be blamed for assuming a *nom de guerre,* realizing early in life that he would be a fighter. But why "Paracelsus"? It is generally held that being highly conceited, Bombastus wished to make it clear that he was superior to Celsus, the chief medical authority of ancient Rome. If that had been so, however, he would have called himself "Hypercelsus." In my opinion "Paracelsus" was chosen to proclaim to the world that he was going to part company with the encyclopedists and methodists in medicine whom Celsus represented, and intended to blaze a new trail by actual experimentation.

In that area, although he made no substantial discoveries, Paracelsus was a pioneer. Had he known enough to consign to the rubbish heap the whimseys which he had accumulated, interweaving them with his sound insights, we might have recognized him as a giant in the field of *materia medica.* Instead he dissipated a great deal of energy combating his colleagues, who naturally did whatever they could to make his life unbearable.

While still a boy, he had the advantage of assisting his father, a physician. Even then he could see through smug verbiage and *ex cathedra* statements which had no basis in fact. Born and bred in what is now German Switzerland, at sixteen, he entered the University of Basel with the intention of becoming a physician, but he soon grew tired of his professors, who merely taught what their predecessors had repeated for centuries. He took to chemistry, which was then little more than alchemy, and, like all chemists of the day, became interested in such chimeras as finding the elixir of life and the philosopher's stone, which would turn the baser metals into gold. Primarily, however, he treated patients, becoming an eminent practitioner sought by the nobility.

While the academically recognized physicians were palming off their fanciful panaceas and concoctions, Paracelsus was bent upon doing genuine field work, experimenting with herbs and drugs to discover their efficacy. So many of the ruling class were among his admirers that he received a call to teach at the University, which he had left without obtaining his medical degree, though he secured it afterward in Italy. In his lectures, he was anything but conventional. Instead of Latin, he held forth in German, which was considered almost a profanation. He emphasized no theory but experience. Definitions, which to the Scholastics were the *sine qua non,* and often the very core, of a subject discussed, were minimized, and the most stress laid on nature. It was evident to Paracelsus that if he went to first sources for his knowledge, his conclusions must be acceptable, while those based on theory alone might or might not be valid.

Had he stated his case more tactfully, he might have incurred the mere jealousy of his colleagues, but his attitude was militant. Like the Prophets of Israel, he was intent upon exposing their ignorance, their insincerity, and their self-complaisance. They, on the other hand, saw in him an erratic, recalcitrant, supercilious, and unacademic interloper, constituting a threat to their sodality.

He was thirty-three when he began teaching at Basel, and after three years as a professor, he was turned out, and his years of vagabondage started. These lasted for twelve years, until the Archbishop of Salzburg befriended and offered him a home. But his substance had already been spent, and he died soon after.

Paracelsus wrote voluminously, but had trouble getting his works published during his lifetime. Occasionally, he astounds us by some observation which sounds psychoanalytic. In his attitude toward the insane, as toward the poor, he reminds us again of the Prophets, who castigated the predatory rich, and pleaded for the underdog.

He set himself up as a commission of one to guard against the unscrupulous methods of apothecaries, who were both careless, exorbitant, and in league with physicians to fleece the patient, although, on the other hand, it may be charged that Paracelsus himself brewed his own medicines for personal gain.

Having been influenced, through secondary and tertiary sources, by Jewish mysticism, he followed the general parallelistic scheme of the Cabbala. The microcosm corresponds to the macrocosm. Diseases will find their antidotes in elements of nature. Basically there are only three types of diseases and three remedies in different combinations, according to the complexity of the ailment. These are salt, sulphur, and mercury, each in two forms. In a sense, his system is homeopathic; and he proposed the naming of a disease according to its remedy, assuming, apparently, that the remedy is known simultaneously with the ailment.

Being steeped in the occult, Paracelsus was bound to seek aid from all sorts of mystic sources. In his *Paramirum* (note how his book titles carry the trademark of his name) he discusses "the origin of invisible diseases." In the *mumia,* or magnetic body, he finds much healing power.

Perhaps his chief work is *On the Greater Surgery,* which passed through many Latin editions, and is said to have been a source book for Ambroise Paré, the father of modern surgery. Paracelsus, who, as his father's assistant, had already received some training in dressing wounds, traveled far and wide to gain further experience, and it was on the battlefields in Europe that he mastered his profession. In *A Book of Defenses,* we are told:

> My travels have developed me: No man becomes a master at home, nor finds his teacher behind the stove. For knowledge is not all locked up, but is distributed throughout the whole world. . . . Sicknesses wander here and there the whole length of the world. . . . If a man wishes to under-

> stand them he must wander too. A doctor must be an alchemist. [We must remember that the term chemistry was not known at the time—A.A.R.] He must, therefore, see the mother earth where the minerals reside, and as the mountains will not come to him he must go to the mountains.

Paracelsus writes with verve and self-assurance. For his students, his forthright utterances must have carried conviction. Speaking of wisdom as an essential in the treatment of disease, he delivers an observation which is valid even today:

> It is true that those who do not seek it [i.e. wisdom] have more wealth than those who do. The doctors who sit by the stove [we should say, in their drawing rooms and Cadillacs] wear chains and silk; those who travel can barely afford a smock. Those who sit by the stove eat partridges and those who follow after knowledge eat milk-soup.

CHARLATAN OR MAN OF SCIENCE?

Four centuries have elapsed since his death, and yet biographers and discussants are still at variance as to his place in the history of medicine. Anna Stoddart has written an illuminating, although perhaps too glowing, account of his life, biased by her own occult learnings.[19] Nevertheless, we must take cognizance of the fact that such an authority as Karl Sudhoff devoted years of his life to examining the authenticity of some of Paracelsus' works, publishing the results in two large volumes.

Jung, who may be looked upon as a modern successor of Paracelsus, thinks that it is virtually impossible to do justice to him. He must be either overrated or underrated. To Jung, he is the prototype of Faust, a "volcanic eruption which disturbed and destroyed but also fructified and vivified." He sees in him a "trail blazer not only of chemical medicine but also of empirical psychology and psychotherapy."[20]

On the other hand, R. M. Lawrence, himself a physician, takes a rather dim view of the man who stirred up the intellectual world of the fifteenth century and who opened the sluice gates that let out streams of impurities but let in waters that were equally foul. However, Lawrence surely exaggerates when he tells us that "Paracelsus was an ignoramus, who affected to despise the sciences because of his lack of knowledge of them. While prating much about divine light as the source of all learning and culture, his boorish mien and rude manners afforded evidence that he did not profit much by its happy influence." [21]

WAR UPON THE DEVIL DELUSION

The Sixteenth century was a period of bedevilment for the civilized portion of Europe, particularly Germany. Stories about witches and their infernal consorts were probably common conversational topics. If anything went wrong, the Devil offered a ready explanation for it. Ordinary diseases might have natural causes, but even here one might apply the phrase, "*Cherchez le diable.*" Mental disorders, because of the abnormal behavior of the sufferers, were definitely attributed to the maleficence of sorcerers and witches, who were the agents, either voluntary or forced, of the Evil One. The very word "maleficence" assumed the sense of "witchcraft" (*maleficium*).

It is evident that under such circumstances, *i.e.*, when the supernatural is alleged to be the source of derangement, and incantations are resorted to as a means of warding off or exorcising the Devil, and the hysteric or schizophrenic is burnt as a witch, no therapy is possible. Since the very first step toward treatment was hindered by such a belief, it was imperative to clear the air of the Devil by showing that the accused witches were mainly sick women. The dragon of mephitic superstition had to be slain before the holy grail of psychiatry could be reached.

That there were professional malefactors, both men and women, who pretended to possess supernatural powers or magical formulae, and who for a consideration would work mischief on an enemy or promise to effect a cure, there can be no doubt. Such mountebanks thrive even in our own day. However, the large majority of the unfortunates to be tortured and executed were harmless eccentrics or psychotics, or perhaps only neurotics.

Who would be their savior, and at the same time pave the way for psychiatry as a science? It was perhaps poetic justice that the protégé of the man most reviled, both alive and dead, by the fanatical sadists should have taken upon himself the mission of enlightening the world. It was Johann Weyer, Agrippa's special student, who shattered the whole superstitious structure obstructing the development of medical psychology, by stifling it *in perpetuum.*

A native of Northern Brabant, and the son of a merchant, Weyer received the usual schooling, and in 1532, at the age of seventeen, he journeyed to Bonn, where Agrippa had found a haven in the court of a German duke, to study with the master. Weyer, although not the sparkling versatile mind that we found Paracelsus to be, was endowed with qualities which served the cause much better. In the first place, he was prudent and well balanced. The ego, which loomed so large in both of his predecessors, was never allowed to mar his writings. Accordingly he received a wider hearing and his words were more effective.

Not having been exposed to the occult, he could concentrate on actual medical cases with the eyes of a professional. Indeed, it may be said of him that he was the first clinical psychiatrist in that he employed modern methods of observation. He resolved on a more or less permanent residence, and spent most of his life happily as court physician to Duke William III of Jülich-Berg-Cleves, whom he would accompany on his travels. Enjoying the protection of a ruler, and naturally guarded in his form of expression, he was able to accomplish far more than the two stormy petrels who had previously aroused the medical world; and being a more patient observer, he made more solid contributions to medicine.

FATHER OF MODERN PSYCHIATRY

Johann Weyer, or Weier, was twenty years old when he lost his mentor, Agrippa, who, three years earlier, had accorded him the hospitality of his house and initiated him into the art of healing. The abuse which befell Agrippa in Germany must have so disgusted the studious youth that he decided to go to France, where the witch obsession did not exercise the hold on the popular mind that it did in Germany under the sway of the Dominicans. Paris, too, was the great center of learning, and its medical faculty was especially noted.

He left Paris for some time, in order to care for the family of the Queen of Navarre at Orléans, but returned to complete his studies and receive his medical diploma.

Among the diseases which he studied and described in great detail, in *Observationes Medicae,* were trichinosis, marsh fever, military (English) sweat, syphilis, scrofula, influenza, occlusion of the cervix, and amenorrhea. Gynecologists are indebted to him for a speculum facilitating vaginal examination.

His *magnum opus,* however, was a work entitled *De Praestigiis Daemonum* (*On the Delusions about Demons*), which he completed in 1562, and published in Basel in 1563. In twenty years, this work went through six editions in Latin, three in German, and two in French. In 1577 (*De Commentitiis Jejuniis*) he gave an account of a simulated fast on the part of a young girl who became something of a celebrity in her town, receiving many gifts from the gullible and testimonials from town officials. Weyer made it his business to examine the ten-year-old girl, and then had the Duke summon the child to Cleves, so he could check up on the claim more scientifically. It transpired that Barbara, as she was called, ate and drank normally, her older sister clandestinely passing her food. The Duke would have penalized the family, but was prevailed upon by the kindhearted physician with a sense of humor to consider the deception only a venial sin. In this experiment, Weyer and his family carried out the investigation much as it would have been done today by a physician, a social worker, a psychiatrist, and perhaps a pastor.

Weyer's two-volume work on demons, which in the lingo of today might be titled "Tomfoolery about Devils," contains more than meets the eye. In the first place, it is a learned book. The author has delved into the subject of witchcraft from all angles. Then, too, he is cautious in the expression of his religious convictions. He does not attempt to brush aside all Biblical references a priori, but dwells on cases which have come to his notice, and which he can diagnose with assurance as those of mental aberration. He does more than that. In carefully describing the symptoms, he affords us glimpses of various types of psychosis; and as he recounts the old wives' tales that had come to his ear, he demonstrates how fantastic they are, and in a humorous vein, exposes the contradictions which would follow from their acceptance, at the same time excoriating the inquisitors and convicting judges for their lack of common sense and their extreme brutality.

In protest against this brutality, he was impelled to write a booklet, *De Irae Morbo* (*On the Disease of Rage*) in which he not only exposes the folly of anger, since much that provokes us is in reality trivial, but appeals to those who have jurisdiction over their fellow-men to temper their hardness and reconsider their sentences.

It would have been a great satisfaction to Agrippa to have seen how his pupil dealt with the devil-mongers, effectually completing the task which he himself had begun so inauspiciously, and realizing perhaps that he had been the stimulus in the shaping of this great work.

Weyer's *De Praestigiis* is a mine of information, touching on different fields. He sometimes introduces his own theories as to why certain phenomena take place. For instance, the nightmare, which had generally been supposed caused by a demon, he explains as a somatic dream, reinforced by the play of imagination while asleep. Other phenomena he explains as the effect of drugs, like hashish, or of excessive suggestibility. He describes depressive as well as manic states, megalomania, paranoia, guilt complexes—all in a lucid and often entertaining style.

What he does is to disabuse the mind of his more intelligent readers—and certainly they had to be educated to read such books—dispelling the mist from before their eyes so that they could judge more realistically. He ransacks history and culls many couplets and quatrains from the poets, both ancient and contemporary, to improve rather than prove his argument. He addresses his readers as if he were a barrister pleading before a judge and jury, all the while aware that some of them will remain immune to reason. He appears to have been familiar with Hebrew and the more important commentators, making fine distinctions, based on etymology, among the various kinds of magic mentioned in the Old Testament.

When it comes to poking fun at the obscurantists, particularly the authors of the notorious *Malleus,* he minces no words and does not leave it to our imagination to interpret his opinion. Citing the tale of the so-called witch who enticed four abbots successively, three of whom, having been served dung and copulated with, died, while the fourth lost his senses, he is disposed to see the events in a different light. To him the alleged witch who the inquisitors bitterly complained was not brought to book (i.e., to the stake to burn) was simply a veteran harlot, while the monks were possessed not by the witch or her master, but by their own lechery, and what she had served them was their wonted and wanted fare, voluptuous ordure which proved a bit too rich for them.[22]

The magic dishes and brews which women prepare, he contends, are natural love charms which they exercise on their lovers. Perfumes and unguents are aids in this art, but can this be called witchcraft?

Without reserve, he relates the rumor about Martin Luther's birth, namely, that one day the Devil, posing as a jewelry salesman, asked for lodging in a middle-class home in Wittenberg, on the ground that it would not be safe for him to stay in an inn. The host, who was well compensated, consented. During the night, the guest, by presents, cajoleries, and other allurements, impregnated the pretty daughter of the house; and the child she brought into the world was the man who stood up to the Catholic Church. He became a monk when he grew up, and having raped a nun, found himself divested of his orders. Having no redress from Rome, he began to undermine the influence of the Church, and in this undertaking received the aid of his "father," who made it easy for him to persuade large bodies of people. He was thus able to dress up his commentaries and orations with such artifices that they appealed not only to the ignorant but to the learned. Weyer, himself a Roman Catholic, asks how one can expect to refute Luther's reformed creed by such scurrilous trash, especially when Luther's biography is so well known and documented?

It was lucky for Weyer that the witch-hunters could not lay their all too eager hands on him. Duke William, his protector, was too powerful. Nevertheless it required courage to gainsay theological and juridical authority, and Weyer must be given credit for his militant stand. He was blunt but not arrogant like his predecessors, and was careful enough to avoid theological controversy. Had the Duke died, it might not have gone well with the crusader; and when a stroke did threaten his life, Weyer was implicated by his foes as the indirect cause of it. Weyer's sudden death in 1588, as he was attending a patient in Tecklenburg, must have been the occasion of great rejoicing in the enemy camp, that this noisome "witch-lover," as they thought of him, was *hors de combat.*

Bodin—Foremost Foe

Such a complex puzzle is human personality that one has difficulty understanding why Jean Bodin (1530-1596), a trained lawyer, celebrated as the founder of political science, as an economist whose service to France was inestimable, and a statesman who championed personal liberty at the risk of falling from royal grace—why this truly liberal spirit should have been Weyer's most implacable adversary and staunchest protagonist of the inquisitors in their witch hunts.

However, Bodin the lawyer was not as enlightened or as far-sighted as Bodin the statesman. He was a firm believer in the Bible, and if Holy Writ tells us there were witches in Biblical times; why should they not still be practicing their nefarious trade? Has the Devil taken a vacation? And as to Weyer's plea on behalf of frail woman, Bodin goes to some length to prove from the Bible that woman is inferior to man (Solomon said that out of a thousand women, not a single decent one could be found). He also quotes Hippocrates, who is reported to have written that women who still possess their virginity do not yield to the various manias; and thus he can well understand why the Devil should be in confederacy with women rather than with men.

Furthermore, by his defense of witches Weyer himself has become an *advocatus diaboli,* in the literal sense; for every witch can claim mental illness. Indeed, since Weyer spoke so highly of Agrippa, even admitting that he often took his master's black poodle out on a leash, that same poodle which was known to have followed Agrippa to the cemetery, disappearing afterward into thin air, what is more likely than the author of *De Praestigiis* is a sorcerer himself?

Amusingly enough, in order to make his point, Bodin confides that since his thirty-seventh year he has been served by a demon, who, on proper invocation, would help him make decisions by touching his left ear when his judgment was good, his right ear when his judgment was poor. Perhaps this demon was nothing but a conditioned itch which developed whenever he was in a quandary, just as some men scratch the back of their heads when in doubt.

To the more charitably inclined, who respected his professional standing, Weyer was simply an egghead who may have been a shark in his own field but who did not understand the ways of the world and the wiles of witches. Weyer did not endure the vilification of Agrippa, but for centuries his epochal work was on the prohibited Index of the Roman Catholic Church. Zilboorg, who devotes nearly forty pages to Weyer in his *History of Medical Psychology,* aptly summarizes his contributions in these words:

> Weyer's contributions can be summarized as follows: He was the first physician whose major interest turned toward mental diseases and thereby foreshadowed the formation of psychiatry as a medical specialty. He was the first clinical and the first descriptive psychiatrist to leave to suc-

ceeding generations a heritage which was accepted, developed, and perfected in an observational branch of medicine in a process which culminated in the great descriptive system of psychiatry formulated at the end of the nineteenth century. Weyer more than anyone else completed, or at least brought closer to completion, the process of divorcing medical psychology from theology and empirical knowledge of the human mind from the faith in the perfection of the human soul. He reduced the clinical problems of psychopathology to simple terms of everyday life and of everyday, human, inner experiences without concealing the complexity of human functioning and the obscurity of human problems.[23]

King James Blasts Scot and Weyer

Bodin wrote his *Démonomanie des Sorciers* in refutation of Weyer in 1580, and in 1584, an Englishman by the name of Reginald Scot, a layman who shared the same humane and enlightened views as the German doctor, published his *Discoverie of Witchcraft,* in sixteen books, in which he punctured general superstitions and decried "the unchristian practices and inhuman dealings of searchers and witch-tryers . . . in extorting confessions by terrors and tortures." Meanwhile books on demonology were appearing in various countries, and schizophrenics were being butchered and burned for asserting the reality of their megalomaniac delusions (emperor, Christ, angel).

If Weyer had the dubious honor of antagonizing a celebrity like Jean Bodin, Scot called down on himself the wrath of a monarch, King James I, who ordered the burning of his book. The King also seized the opportunity to display his literary gifts by refuting Scot, whom he mentions, with Weyer, in his *Daemonologie,* published in 1597. At the very opening of the book, we are able to catch a glimpse of the temper in England toward the end of the sixteenth century.

> The fearful abounding at this time in this country of the detestable slaves of the devil, the witches or enchanters, hath moved me, beloved reader, to despatch in post this following treatise of mind, not in anywise, as I protest, to serve for a show of my learning and ingine, but only, moved of conscience, to press thereby, so far as I can, to resolve the doubting hearts of many; both that such assaults of Sathan are most certainly practised, and that the instruments thereof merits [*sic*] most severely to be punished: against the damnable opinions of two principally in our age, whereof the one called Scot, an Englishman, is not ashamed in public print to deny that there can be such a thing as witchcraft; and so maintains the old error of the Sadducees in denying of spirits. The other called Wierus, a German physician, sets out a public apology for all these crafts-folks, whereby, procuring for their impunity, he plainly betrays himself to have been one of that profession. And for to make this treatise the more pleasant and facile, I have put it in form of a dialogue, which I have divided into three books: the first speaking of magic in general, and necromancy in special; The second, of sorcery and witchcraft; and the third contains a discourse of all these kinds of spirits and spectres that appears [*sic*] and troubles persons; together with a conclusion of the whole work.

Notwithstanding, the natural approach to mental disease was beginning to prevail in France as well as in England. François Bayle (1622-1709) (not to be confused with Pierre Bayle, the skeptic), teaching at the University of Toulouse discarded such notions as lunar influences as a cause of menstruation, the pineal gland as the seat of the soul (Descartes), the still flickering dogma of demoniac possession, and looked to the nervous system for explanations of insanity. In some of his works he urges a co-operative study among the physical scientists, physicians, and surgeons, thus indicating a progressive trend.

ST. VINCENT DE PAUL (1576-1660)
Savior of the Handicapped

A native of Gascony, of humble birth, Vincent de Paul was brought up by Franciscan monks and ordained in 1600. Captured by pirates while sailing along the French coast, he was sold as a slave in Tunis. Converting one of his masters, an Italian, he made his way with him to France where he functioned as a curate, then as a tutor to the children of Count de Joigney, in the vicinity of Amiens. Wherever he sojourned he made devoted friends, endearing himself especially to the lowly. Peasants and titled ladies alike fell in with his suggestions, and so the ramified system of benevolent societies and missions, which today are known by his name, came into being.

It must be borne in mind that four hundred years ago, the unfortunate were left to their own devices. Occasionally a prince, a countess, or a high ecclesiastic would make some contribution toward the assuaging of misery among the wretched, generally social outcasts, but it was thanks to Vincent de Paul's energy and devotion, his empathy rather than sympathy with the underprivileged, that the Bicêtre, originally a castle which belonged to the Bishop of Winchester, was founded as the great French asylum. Later some of the funds which Vincent de Paul had collected were diverted to the founding of the still more famous Salpêtrière, where psychiatric history was made by such men as Pinel, Esquirol, and Charcot. De Paul's labors on behalf of the suffering included establishing a hospital for galley slaves (Marseille), a sisterhood for charity, two homes for foundlings, and a junior sisterhood to minister to the sick and the poor. Pope Clement XII canonized him in 1737. His life has been told by Maynard in four volumes.

Stahl—First Modern Vitalist

One of the men of the early eighteenth century who have been receiving more attention in our own century is Georg Ernst Stahl (1694-1734). Called to fill the chair of medicine at the newly founded University of Halle, he afterward became physician to the King of Prussia (Friedrich Wilhelm), following him to Berlin. The man who sponsored Stahl was Friedrich Hoffmann, himself a noted authority, who was carried away by the physiological and chemical discoveries that were making medical history. Apparently Stahl, too, was greatly influenced by the chemical, physical, and physiological theories of medicine, but he soon broke away from his sponsor and began to propagate a vitalistic doctrine, even going so far as to attribute every type of activity to the soul.

In a letter to Schroeck, he speaks of the absurdity of attributing all kinds of diseases to the acridity of the humors. If the humors continue to deteriorate, then suppuration and gangrene should set in. Although brought up on the respectable principles of Sylvius and Willis, Stahl could no longer accept the view that a certain mixture, chemical or other, could produce life and initiate a complexity of function.

The odd thing was that Stahl did some outstanding research in chemistry. It was he who, in conjunction with Becher, propounded the theory that combustion takes place as a result of the separation of phlogiston from a given substance—a theory which held sway for a full century, until Lavoisier showed that the element involved was oxygen, and that the hypothetical phlogiston was a chimera.

Stahl, however, was not the first scientist to lean toward what may be considered its opposite pole. Among physicists and astronomers one may name Zöllner, Crookes, Oliver Lodge, and Flammarion; while the physiologists Sherrington and Cannon repudiate behavioristic explanations, even rejecting the James-Lange theory of emotions; and Freud, specializing in neurology, ignores all physiology in working out the psychoanalytic system.

Stahl's "soul" is simply the sum-total of the non-material side of man and animals, which, together with nature, can effect the desired cure, often regardless of the state of the body. The soul can err, too, and here Stahl differentiates the *logos* and the *logismos,* through both of which the soul performs its functions.[24] In modern terms, we might call the former *reason,* the second *rationalization.* It is because animals do not rationalize, but are led by their instinct, that there is less disease among them, and less still among wild animals than among the domestic, which have taken over some human foibles.

Stahl is an interactionist, in that he thinks the mind affects the body, just as the body affects the mind, although in the last analysis the mind rules. The emotions and habits play a very important part in the bringing on or staving off of disease. Hence, reason and will power should be considered to a greater degree than humors or drugs.

For several reasons Stahl did not gain the wide hearing his works should have commanded. In the first place, his Latin style was awkward and involved. Secondly, he was moving against the current. Physiology was considered at the time the palladium of all medicine and neurology the answer to all mental ills. For a man to pooh-pooh the hard-won achievements of the laboratories was thought to be a sign of failing mentality. In addition, Stahl, reminiscent of Paracelsus and Agrippa (although he did not share their mysticism and flare for the occult), criticized with considerable vehemence colleagues who had attained eminent status, while displaying considerable arrogance and egocentricity in the promulgation of his own views.

Once we substitute "psyche" for "soul" and recognize the force that the emotions (affects) exert on everyday activities, often bottling up our executive impulses, we can see that Stahl was looking toward a dynamic interpretation of behavior and its deviations. Because of the stress he laid on the affective life, which ran counter to the German trend, we can also understand why his views were honored in France rather than in Germany.

No less a philosopher and scientist than the great Leibniz was Stahl's chief antagonist, and carried on an extended controversy with him. Leibniz accused Stahl of materialism because he chose to believe that body and mind interacted directly instead of agreeing with Leibniz's doctrine of pre-established harmony through the wisdom and beneficence of God. Stahl was a religious man, but he did not care to become a theologian or a metaphysician. Had he lived today, he might well have belonged to some school of depth psychology which puts a premium on self-discipline and moral behavior.

In Zilboorg's opinion, Stahl was the originator of the distinction between organic and functional mental disease.[25] For the first time, it was set forth that mental disorders are the result of neither physical, mechanical, nor supernatural forces, but are psychogenic, or at least biogenic, in origin.

Langermann Founds First German Mental Hospital

One of the followers of Stahl during the eighteenth century was J. G. Langermann (1768-1832), who wrote the first doctoral dissertation on psychiatry, in

1797, under the title *On the Method of Diagnosing and Treating Chronic Mental Diseases.* In this thesis, which was naturally in Latin, he made an attempt to go further than Stahl, maintaining that a physical disease may often be due to psychic causes. Thus Langermann is entitled to a place among the pioneers of psychosomatic medicine, as well as of psychotherapy.

Another distinction which should be credited to him is that he was the first to found a mental hospital in Germany, in 1805. It was named St. Georg, and was located in the little Franconian town of Bayreuth. Unlike most of his medical countrymen and the great English physicians of the time, Langermann was sympathetically inclined toward the unfortunate inmates of his hospital, which he directed for five years, and treated the insane with tenderness and understanding. To him they were people and not outcasts. Without turning out hefty treatises and textbooks, he exercised a deep influence over some of his brilliant students, who were later to become pre-eminent themselves.

ROBERT BURTON—
The Encyclopedist of Melancholy

Robert Burton was a clergyman and attic scholar, whose *Anatomy of Melancholy* (1621) became one of the monuments of English literature, and was a best-seller for years, reaping a fortune for its publishers. The poem which prefaces the book is a gem in itself, and its simple refrain, "Naught so sweet as melancholy," "so sour," "so sad," "so damned," served Milton as a model in the writing of *Il Penseroso* and of one of his masques.

Burton was given to chronic depression, and therefore his own introspective account contains a wealth of observation, but he also recorded the behavior of others whom he suspected of moodiness; and probably no one before him so thoroughly plowed the world's literature for material on assorted eccentricities and whimseys. The great volume, for all its rambling and frequent irrelevancies as well as inaccuracies, makes fascinating reading even today.

Burton, who is said to have calculated the date of his death and made sure that his calculation was right, covers his subject from A to Z, making melancholy a universal disease. In his introduction ("Democritus to the Reader") he asks rhetorically, "Indeed who is not a fool, melancholy, mad?—Who attempts nothing foolish, who is not brain-sick? Folly, melancholy, madness, are all but one disease." Does he not agree, then, with the psychoanalysts? And if he puts all his fish in one kettle, he can afterward begin sorting them in his own sweet way, by stringing authorities together. He does distinguish between melancholy and madness, corresponding to our dichotomy of neurosis and psychosis. Another rather modern aperçu is "No man can cure himself" (*Part I, Sect.* 1, *Memb.* 1). His classification is topographical: head, heart, and hepatic; and one leads to the other. "For our body is like a clock; if one wheel be amiss, all the rest are disordered."

He is not prepared to take sides on the part each of the humors (blood, phlegm, yellow bile, and black bile in the Galenian scheme) plays in the various types nor on the role of the Devil and demons, but he presents the opinions of scores of writers via their cock-and-bull stories. However, to play safe, he includes the spirits, that is, demons, as one cause of melancholy—with God's permission, of course. We must look to wizards and witches for another cause. And how can we ignore the stars and their influences, though "if we are ruled by reason, they have no power over us"? Considering the millions even in our educated country who take stock in the newspaper horoscope, and read the astrology magazines, we can scarcely blame Burton, born nearly four centuries ago, for his superstitions.

Other causes of disorder he adduces seem more sensible, such as old age (involutional dementia), heredity, bad diet, constipation, continence or sexual excesses, bad air, idleness, solitariness, overexcitement ("perturbations of mind"), overplay of imagination, fears, shame and disgrace, envy, malice, hatred, emulation, anger, discontents, miseries, immoderate pleasures—but why enumerate them all? It suffices to observe that in some respects he hit the nail on the head; and his anecdotes add spice rather than proof. If psychoanalysts believe that Freud was the first to associate neurosis with sex, then let them read what Burton has to say:

> Felix Plater, in the first Book of His Observations, tells a story of an ancient Gentleman in Alsatia, that married a young wife, and was not able to pay his debts in that kind for a long time together, by reason of his several infirmities: but she, because of this inhibition of Venus, fell into a horrible fury, and desired every one that came to see her, by words, looks, and gestures, to have to do with her, etc. Bernardus Paternus, a physician saith, he knew a good honest godly Priest, that, because he would neither willingly marry, nor make use of the stews, fell into a grievous melancholy fits. Wildesheim hath such another example of an Italian melancholy Priest in a consultation had in the year 1580. Jason Pratensis gives instance in a married man, that from his wife's death abstaining, after marriage, became exceeding melancholy.[26]

A confirmed bachelor and probably ascetic throughout life, he was familiar with all the stratagems of love, and that part of his book might serve as a fitting propaedeutic to Havelock Ellis' *Psychology of Sex*. In the section on "Remedies of Love," he certainly, without terming it so, expounds the dynamic concept of sublimation, so significant as a mechanism in psychoanalysis.

The Situation in British Medical Circles

Robert Burton's *Anatomy of Melancholy* made delightful reading, but it made no dent in the course of mental pathology, for one reason because its author was not a medical man. England could boast of great names in medicine, even in the early part of the seventeenth century. William Harvey made his great discovery of the circulation of the blood in 1619, although he did not publish his well-established theory until 1628. About mid-century, Thomas Sydenham, who was sometimes referred to as the English Hippocrates, developed the notion that every disease is the consequence of a progressive pathological process, which he took pains, in his practice, to investigate thoroughly. Yet mental disease seemed too intangible a field for the empirical Englishmen to tackle. On the Continent, Felix Plater (1536-1614), whom Burton cites frequently, made at least an attempt to examine mental patients with a view to classifying their disorders. Not that he was farther advanced in his views than the non-professional Burton, but his interest was patient-centered, that is to say, he dealt with them even if he did not understand them. Charles Lepois (1563-1633) devoted chapters of a medical textbook to hysteria, which he thought had nothing to do with the womb, as had been commonly believed since the days of Hippocrates.

English therapists applied mostly a crude shock treatment. Thus Thomas Willis (1621-1675), who discovered the Willis circle in the cerebral arteries and declared the process of respiration one of combustion, took an otiose attitude to the insane, recommending punishment for failure to exercise control—a method just the reverse of that prescribed by the humane Agrippa and Weyer in the previous century. One often wonders whether empathy is a quality possessed by capable researchers.

The Scottish practitioner and Edinburgh professor, William Cullen (1710-1790), was perhaps not so original a researcher, but his standing in Europe was greater than that of Willis. His book on methods of nosology passed through many Latin editions. Some of his other works were translated into French, German, and Italian. One of the translations was made by Pinel.

His division of diseases into four great classes—(a) fevers, (b) neuroses, (c) habit diseases, like scurvy, and (d) local ones, such as cancer—seems to have made some impression on the medical world, two hundred years ago, although some diseases presented problems of overlapping. He may be regarded as the leader, if not the founder, of the neuropathological school. His critical sense was more developed than his imaginative powers. He recognized the distinctness of sensory and motor nerves, and in place of the antiquated humors, he *attributed the causes of mental disorders to the nervous system.* In speaking of the "nervous fluid," he was, no doubt, referring to the "nerve impulse" of modern textbooks.

John Brown (1735-1788), the founder of what afterward was labeled the Brunonian System, was one of the most picturesque and most controversial characters in the annals of British medicine.

A prodigy who, before he reached the age of ten, had been put to a trade by his stepfather in Scotland, he managed to return to school, and at the age of twenty-five began his medical course at Edinburgh, obtaining leave from the various professors to attend their lectures without paying tuition. He completed his studies, but because of his bohemian tendencies, carefree manner, and flair for rubbing his superiors the wrong way, did not receive his degree at Edinburgh, but was successful at St. Andrews.

He had already gotten into difficulties with his teacher and benefactor, Cullen, and when a formal break took place, Brown began to expose the errors of Cullen's teaching, formulating a new system in a book (*Elementa Medicinae*) which attracted many readers on the Continent, partly because of his finished Latin style. After his death this work was translated into many European languages, and controversies broke out in several countries over its merits.

John Brown did away with the old blood-letting cures and developed, probably from Cullen's cues, a theory that the weakened state of he tissues (cells) was responsible for mental deterioration.

Neurologist Johann Reil Founds First Psychiatric Journal

In Germany, perhaps the most conspicuous early work in linking physiology with psychiatry is associated with the name of Johann C. Reil (1759-1813), a name known to every elementary student of psychology and physiology because of the island in the brain (The island of Reil) which he described so minutely. He is best known as an anatomist and physiologist, but he also functioned as an oculist, a surgeon, and a clinical psychiatrist.

His researches on the nerves (*De Structura Nervorum*), published in 1786, gave him an international reputation, and his founding of the *Archiv f. Physiologie,* followed by his founding, with Kayssler, of the *Magazin f. psychische Heilkunde,* the first psychiatric periodical, points to the prodigiousness of his labors and the scope of his interests.

After fruitful years as a professor at Halle, where he had received his M.D., he went to Berlin as chief clinician, and died in his fifty-fifth year as a result of typhus contracted in the course of his duties at a military hospital. It is an irony of fate that the man who had made the most thorough study of fever, in five volumes, should have been taken by this disease.

Reil taught that energy expresses the relation of certain phenomena to the properties of matter. Every organ, therefore, has its own peculiar irritability and disposition to disease. In this way, he showed a tendency toward decentralization in the understanding of pathological conditions.

Like his colleagues in England, he set great store by the physiological findings of the day, but in his "Rhapsodies on the application of psychic therapy methods to mental disturbances" (1803) he brought to the attention of practitioners the necessity of introducing psychotherapy. What he advocated was a sort of psychodrama in which not the patients but the hospital personnel would act out a sort of tribunal representing celestial personnel, in order to arouse the patients from their lethargy. This may seem bizarre to us, but the pre-enactment of what might happen to them in the next world might have the effect of shock therapy.

In Germany, he was regarded as the *father of psychotherapy*. His was not merely the theoretical or research mind. He carried his message on the amelioration of the condition of the insane to the authorities, suggesting the appointment to mental hospitals of men who were connected with medical schools, deploring the neglect of patients and the inferior quality of the hospitals' administration and staff.

AN EVENTFUL DECADE

Madmen Relieved; Normals Terrorized in Paris

We now approach the nineteenth century. The demoniac delusion had petered out, at least among the physicians and clergy, and with the awakening of the social conscience, as the masses began to assert themselves, particularly in England and in France, sporadic appeals to treat the mentally disturbed more mercifully—appeals which were once voices crying in the desert—were now being heard.

It is often stated that our large hospitals for the insane are neglectful of their inmates, allowing them to vegetate without supplying the individual care needed to relieve the stress and distress, but the plight of the insane two hundred years ago was worse than that of vermin. Kept either in cellar-dungeons or in *Narrentürme* (lunatic towers), they were practically swimming in filth, beaten, shackled, bled, purged frequently, and ducked in almost freezing pools in order to "bring them to their senses." Pigs were treated better, and their styes were far cleaner than the habitats of the mentally ill. It would, indeed, be almost impossible for them to recover after inhabiting such a universe. Those who were still at large were subjected to the raillery of adults and the sadistic tendencies of teen-agers. They were buffeted, kicked, and pelted.

About 180 years ago, Jean Colombier (1736-1789), on the staff of the Hôtel-Dieu in Paris, raised his voice on behalf of the deranged patients. In Italy,

Vincenzo Chiarugi (1759-1820), medical director of the Bonifacio Asylum in Florence, not only preached better treatment for the mentally ill, but put his preachments into practice.

Chiarugi, in a work published in 1794, attempted a classification of mental diseases, according to cause, diagnosis, prognosis, and treatment. Pinel, who commended Chiarugi for his observations, and especially for his initiative in lifting asylum inmates out of their miserable depths, nevertheless did not think much of his system, calling it scholastic rather than empirical.

Things were beginning to look up for psychotics when Joseph Daquin, an older contemporary of Pinel, in Paris voiced thoughts similar to Chiarugi's, converting them into action at the hospital in Chambéry, of which he had charge. But before telling his story, we must turn to England.

A Quaker Merchant to the Rescue

It has already been noted that the celebrated physicians in England were mind-ruled rather than affected by the heart, and guided by tradition whenever they could not resort to empirical research. Neither Sydenham, nor Cullen, nor Willis could muster the feeling that was required to break completely with the past, although Willis did declare himself for humane treatment, and served his mental patients better than his predecessors.

It took a prosperous Quaker by the name of William Tuke (1732-1822) to right the wrongs which physicians only condemned in their books. The revolting abuse of the mentally disturbed in the York Asylum so affected him that he addressed himself to a number of his fellow members of the Society of Friends, and with their assistance, in 1792, established the York Retreat. Tuke lived to the ripe age of ninety, so that he devoted some three decades to the reform of the treatment of mental patients, thus setting an example for others. Both his son Henry and his grandson Samuel, neither of whom was a physician, dedicated themselves to the task of expanding and improving the York Retreat, which became a model for similar institutions in England and the United States.

The York Retreat was a haven for the most abject creatures, coming from their cellar-dungeons. For Tuke it was not a retreat but a great advance. More than a century of far-sighted philanthropy was initiated by this Quaker tea merchant, whose great-grandson, James, was instrumental in bringing succor to starving Ireland, through his intercession with the members of parliament, while another great-grandson, Daniel Hack Tuke (1827-1895) ranked as one of England's best-trained and most benign alienists, as psychiatrists were then called. He was the most representative British medical man of his day—a leader at international meetings, and reminding us of William James—dignified in appearance, genteel and benign in his relations with people.

Among his works, *Insanity in Ancient and Modern Literature, History of the Insane in the British Isles, A Dictionary of Medical Psychology* and, with J. C. Bucknill as co-author, *A Manual of Psychological Medicine* were highly thought of, while his best-known treatise, *Illustrations on the Influence of Mind on Body,* probably gave rise to the oft-heard phrase, "the power of mind over body."

His *Dictionary of Medical Psychology* was a tremendous enterprise, in two large volumes. The first of its kind on a comprehensive scale, it numbered among its contributors some of the greatest authorities in the world—a truly international group, with Charcot as its most noted name.

What conditions were like at the oldest and chief asylum in England, which everyone knows as Bedlam (originally Bethlehem), may be gleaned from the description an unwelcome reformer, who forced his way into the Hospital in 1814, gave before the Committee of the House of Commons.

> In the women's galleries, one of the side rooms contained about ten patients, each chained by one arm or leg to the wall, the chain allowing them merely to stand up by the bench or form fixed to the wall, or to sit down on it. The nakedness of each patient was covered by a blanket, made into something like a dressing-gown, but with nothing to fasten it in front. This was the whole covering, the feet being naked. In another part he found many of the unfortunate women locked up in their cells, naked, and chained on straw, with only one blanket for a covering. In the men's wing, in the side room, six patients were chained close to the wall, five handcuffed and one locked to the wall by the right arm, as well as by the right leg; he was very noisy; all were naked except as to the blanket-gown or small rug on the shoulders, and without shoes—their nakedness and their mode of confinement gave this room the complete appearance of a dog-kennel.
>
> In one of the cells of the lower gallery we saw William Norris. He stated himself to be fifty-five years of age, and that he had been confined about fourteen years; that in consequence of attempting to defend himself from what he conceived the improper treatment of his keeper, he was fastened by a long chain, which, passing through a partition, enabled the keeper, by going into the next cell, to draw him close to the wall at pleasure.[27]

No wonder the word "Bedlam" came to denote, in common parlance, the depths of squalor and raving madness—a synonym of pandemonium. Even Hogarth's portrayals in his *Rake's Progress* series hardly convey a true picture of conditions there, which persisted as late as the nineteenth century.

Pinel Breaks the Chains

The term *fin de siècle* had a sort of existentialist connotation even before Kierkegaard came on the scene, but for the demented confined in public institutions, the last decade of the eighteenth century ushered in a new era—in Italy because of Vincenzo Chiarugi, in England at the York Retreat, but principally in France through Philippe Pinel.

It is interesting that while heads of the aristocracy were rolling off the guillotine, it was in the very institution where this death apparatus had first been tried out on corpses of its inmates, that the mentally ill, the scum and dregs of humanity, as they were regarded by even the Parisian underdogs, were released from their iron fetters. It took courage for Philippe Pinel (1745-1826) to carry out his reforms despite the double hazard which threatened him; for, on the one hand, a madman "on the loose" might very well wreak vengeance for his years of horrible suffering, and on the other, the changing temper of the violent revolutionaries, many of whom were not far removed from those confined as lunatics, could place the rational revolutionary in jeopardy. Nevertheless, Pinel inscribed his name in the book of history by taking the bold step, in 1793, of removing the chains from his Bicêtre charges.

We are indebted to Pinel's great-grandnephew, R. Semelaigne, for a graphic account of the circumstances which finally culminated in this act of mercy. Pinel was inclined to take the revolutionary step almost immediately on entering the institution as director, but he was advised that permission would have to be gained from the Commune. Pinel went before the Commune and made a fervent plea before the head of the Convention, the impetuous Georges Couthon, who the following year (1794) was borne to the scaffold in the same cart as his staunch friend, Robespierre.

Couthon, seeing danger for the Revolution on all sides, sternly warned the physician that if he intended to protect some of the enemies of the people (how familiar the phrase still sounds!) he would rue the day. Able executive that he was, despite his paralytic condition, Couthon interrogated some of the fettered psychotics, receiving vile abuse for answers. Turning to Pinel, he exclaimed, "Citizen, you must be crazy yourself to wish to let these brutes loose." Pinel retorted that those deprived of air and liberty could hardly be expected to treat their captors with better grace. Couthon finally left the decision to Pinel, not, however, without predicting that he would regret his foolhardiness.

Pinel did not unfetter the inmates all at once, but gradually, waiting to observe the results in a dozen cases. One of the men he released, a sturdy former soldier, who had tried to pass himself off as a general, had been confined in the asylum for ten years. This man, Chevigné, whom Pinel treated kindly, actually saved his life, when an incited mob, under the delusion that the doctor had been harboring some of the bourgeoisie, was about to lynch him.

How did Pinel himself feel about the experiment? In the preface to his principal work, he writes: "I have examined with scrupulous care the effects which the iron chains had on the insane, and afterward the comparative results of their removal, and I cannot help favoring a wiser and more moderate restraint." [28] He tells of a number of violent cases, who, once the chains were removed, became relaxed and conversed agreeably; and who when they felt it necessary, asked to be strait-jacketed.

At Bicêtre, Pinel instituted a regimen which was free from the insensate bloodletting, purging, and ducking that were the common treatment of the day. As a practicing physician, in his earlier days, he had familiarized himself with French, German, British, and Italian theories and practices, having translated Cullen's *Institutions of Medicine* and Baglivi's *Opera Omnia,* and he was thus fully equipped to undertake the task of hospital administration.

In 1795, when he became the chief of La Salpêtrière, a more modern institution, he was able to carry out all his projects. Due to a succession of brilliant men who followed in his footsteps, culminating in the combined medical skill and showmanship exercised by that towering personality, J-M. Charcot, this hospital remained for a century the psychiatric center of the world, to which flocked almost every aspiring medical graduate in the mental diseases, just as Leipzig was the proving-ground for experimental psychologists.

The term "medico-philosophical" in the title of Pinel's book indicates the author's disagreement with the purely physical remedies everywhere in vogue. He was sympathetic to, and, in fact, respected some of the British medical men and their methods, particularly Willis, but deprecated the callous intellectualistic attitude of the Germans, referring to their practices as "*méthodes gothiques.*"

His treatise on mental alienation is by no means monumental. It is written in a plain, matter-of-fact style, which is accessible to the intelligent layman. He classifies mental diseases according to symptoms, discusses many individual cases, and outlines the course of treatment, which was more along the lines of diet, encouragement, and the lessening of retraint —in general, psychotherapy.

Throughout the book, he points out the dubiousness of the theories advanced by continental practitioners, both his predecessors and contemporaries. Hypotheses were not to his liking. Detailed description of the patient's behavior—a tendency observed in

French medical literature to this day—was to him the *sine qua non* of all treatment. His chief interest, is to spot the symptoms; and in his other noted book, *Nosographie Philosophique*, which served as a standard text, running through many editions, he dealt especially with diagnosis. His classification, considering its time, was based on common sense. His criticism of Cullen and others is, as a rule, well taken.

Pinel's arrangement of rooms and services reveals an engineering type of mind. His careful records, his follow-ups, his coming close to patients in order to understand their inner trouble—all indicate an exceptional therapist. His influence over his students at the University, his uncommon energy, even in his seventh decade, his personal dignity, to the point of never currying favor with the mighty, and his carrying out his resolutions during a revolution when the slightest misstep might have led to the guillotine, set him in a class by himself in the annals of modern psychiatry. One of his outstanding traits was his faith in at least the potential recovery of most of his patients. As a clinician he probably stands second to none in the eighteenth century.

Although Pinel came of a medical family, he did not become interested in medicine until one of his friends went insane, and in his wanderings became the prey of wolves.

To what extent Pinel trusted his intuition and contravened accepted practice is shown by his appointment of Jean-Baptiste Pussin, a former patient and untrained, as supervisor over the men. Pussin, who went with Pinel to Salpêtrière, turned out to be successful in dealing with patients, a natural psychotherapist, whom Pinel publicly commended.

Esquirol—The Hospital Designer

Jean-Etienne-Dominique Esquirol (1772-1840) did nothing quite so spectacular as Pinel's striking off the irons in the asylum. Nevertheless, his name will be remembered as one of the greatest clinicians and hospital designers of the century.

Esquirol left the St. Sulpice Seminary, when the Revolution made his services as a field medical assistant peremptory, in order to study medicine, and was fortunate in becoming the student, and later the assisant of Pinel at Salpêtrière. Pinel found in him a worthy successor, who adopted the master's program, adding to it important measures of his own.

A genial intellectual in appearance, he rose as an administrator step by step. In 1823, he became chief inspector of the University of Paris, and later took over the direction of the large asylum at Charenton.

Like Pinel, he was independent and outspoken when it was a question of helping the cause of humanity. One of the first to point out that the criminally insane should be treated as suffering from disease, he recommended improving the lot of prisoners. Perhaps his greatest triumph came when, as a guest of the Italian King, who proudly showed him around a new asylum, he was bold enough to point out basic flaws which the wise king took under advisement, and turning the asylum into an armory, ordered a new one built incorporating Esquirol's recommendations.

An extremely busy administrator and consultant, he still found time to give courses in psychiatry and to write articles as well as a textbook, which for decades held first place in French institutions. In *Maladies Mentales* (1838), his most important work, he did much to clarify certain issues. He differentiated between hallucinations and illusions, so that the latter would not be associated with mental disorders. He emphasized certain environmental and age (puberty)-precipitating factors, and stressed the study of the emotions in the understanding of mental disease. A number of his articles in the *Dictionnaire des Sciences Médicales* are authoritative monographs in important phases of the field. The statistical bent of

Pinel, in the classification of inmates according to symptoms, factors involved, age, etc., was accentuated by his brilliant pupil. This type of survey laid the foundation for the later care in preparing hospital records as an avenue to the understanding of mental etiology.

FALRET'S MIXING POLICY

Jean-Pierre Falret (1794-1870) might be called a grand-pupil of Pinel, for he was one of Esquirol's outstanding students, who continued the tradition of his predecessors at La Salpêtrière.

Falret made special studies in connection with suicidal tendencies. What he tried to do was to worm his way into the patient's mind, to draw him out by a gentle approach and skillful questioning. Mental hygiene is the field he was actually cultivating, although the term was not coined until much later. The legal and lay attitude toward mental disease was repugnant to him; and like his predecessors, he was constantly at odds with the juridical point of view. The introduction of the term "mental alienation" in place of "dementia" and "furor" was due largely to his efforts. Like Esquirol, he traveled extensively, particularly in the British Isles.

It was Falret who gave the first impetus to considering mania and depression as stages or phases of the same disorder, which he called "folie circulaire." About half a century later, this view was definitely established by Kraepelin and consolidated in the term "manic-depressive psychosis."

The "Belgian Pinel"

Joseph Guislain (1797-1860) deserves to be placed alongside Pinel and Esquirol. A Belgian, he might be looked upon as an intellectual and temperamental descendant of Weyer. What Pinel did in Bicêtre and La Salpêtrière a generation earlier, Guislain performed perhaps even with greater success at Ghent; for he had the manacles removed from the patients' hands and introduced humane treatment, taking an interest in each individual case. The title "liberator of the insane" has often been applied to him as well as to Pinel.

As professor of philosophy and mental disease at the University of Ghent, he wielded great influence over his students. His thirty-nine lectures on what he termed "mental alienation" were careful and specific discussions of all that pertained to psychopathology, empirically treated. He did not go into theory, but followed rather the French tradition of attending to the business of therapy. His observations are nevertheless at times quite arresting. He questions the benefits of frequent visits by relatives, especially women, whose behavior is disturbing to patients. The function of priests in an asylum is outlined judiciously. The various "phrenopathies," as he designates the neuroses and psychoses, are classified much after the French fashion, for example, anxiety states, misanthropic melancholy, demonophobia, erotic melancholy, religious mania; and he alludes to the circularity of violence and sorrow, which suggests the later nomenclature of Kraepelin.[29]

From an administrative angle, he advises not housing patients of the same type together. Herding together all the melancholics only aggravates their state because of the aggregate depression. Again, the apathetic, if brought together in one ward, inhibit each other, so that stark inaction is the result. By the same token, the violent are constantly at war with each other. He therefore suggests grouping them in the hospital, so that, by living together, they can balance one another's defects, and exercise a beneficial influence over one another.[30]

Mixing the patients in this manner, however, does

not mean that the various stages of the disturbances are ignored. On the contrary, different locations are suggested for (a) the convalescent, (b) the peaceable, (c) the disturbed and noisy, (d) the destructive and suicidal, (e) epileptics and idiots, (f) the soilers, who are helpless as regards control over natural functions, and (g) children.

In the second volume, he takes up details of hospital arrangement, lighting, heating, baths; and strikes a middle course between somatic methods and psychotherapy. The latter can be overdone, he thinks, probably with an eye in the direction of his French colleagues. He does take account of specific medications.

In his books,[31] the nervous system receives a good deal of attention. It was not for nothing that he founded the Society of Medicine at Ghent, and served as its first President, but he was not a child of the French Revolution. As a professor of philosophy at the University, he must have moved in an ethico-religious atmosphere. Hence, after his exposition of the nervous system, he goes on to say that it is not so much the nervous system itself that is at the root of the trouble, but that the source is more deep-lying and mystical. It is not difficult to guess that he has the soul in mind. But a more articulate spokesman of the religious point of view in psychiatry was the German, Heinroth.

Sin and Sanity

While the clinical attitude was gaining ground, especially in France, and the neurological school was making headway in both England and Germany, a prospect appeared which seemed more like a reversion to the period when theology and religion dominated the whole range of human experience. This was, of course, a reaction to the inroads of an aggressive somatology, and at the time it was an audacious move not only to reintroduce the concept of a soul into the sphere of mental disease but to connect mental suffering with sin. It was Johann Christian Heinroth (1773-1843) who took the bold step of proclaiming the relationship.

Heinroth was the son of a Leipzig surgeon, who was apparently expected to follow his father's profession. He accompanied a Russian invalid Count to Italy, and when his patient died, Heinroth turned to theology, in which he received a good grounding. Though he never functioned as a clergyman, it may be said that he remained a pastor all his life, returning to medicine and specializing in those diseases which, to his thinking, were linked with the soul.

If Heinroth was a contemporary of Esquirol, who left religion severely alone, he was also a contemporary of Schelling, Schlegel and other romanticists in philosophy, so that he was not really isolated, even if these men were a bit remote from his domain of psychiatry. Wilhelm Hegel, the spiritualist in philosophy, was poaching on abnormal psychology when in his *Phenomenologie des Geistes* he acquaints us with miscellaneous types of what we would call today "nervous breakdowns."

Though Heinroth was ridiculed by the majority of his scientific contemporaries, later para-Freudian trends, the pastoral psychology movement, and even the dissident schools of Jung and Adler have, to some extent, confirmed the premise that there is a tie-up between neurosis and defective character, and that some unitary principle in the individual, rather than the impairment of a particular organ, is involved in mental disorder.

Had Heinroth followed that tack, he would have been less railed at by his colleagues. However, he took a more extreme stand and displayed the zeal of a missionary, operating with terms like "soul" and "sin," which the alienists of the day were intent on keeping out of their science; and he could not help injecting mysticism in a large part of his chief work, *Lehrbuch der Störungen des Seelenlebens* (1818). In reality, he was merely eager to prove the thesis that a Don Juan came to grief in the long run as a result of the guilt that was building up in his psyche. He was in agreement with the Psalmist who begins his masterpiece with the words: "Blessed is the man that walketh not in the counsel of the wicked . . . and he shall be like a tree planted by the rivers of water that bringeth forth his fruit in season; his leaf also shall not wither and whatever he doeth shall prosper."

Once we dispose of Heinroth's propaganda, there is still a great deal of value in his textbook, such as the attempt to classify a host of mental diseases, and his shrewd clinical conclusions. His attitude toward patients was humane, and his efforts on behalf of the criminally insane, described in his *System der psychischgerichtlichen Medizin,* were not without salutary results. That he was a man of many interests is evident from the fact that in one volume he surveyed the basic failures in education and indulged in literary work under a pen name.

Heinroth was not a pure mystic or romantic, but a practical man as well. Through his religious impulse, he became the spearhead of a school that opposed a mechanistic approach toward the understanding and treatment of the insane.

The Father of American Psychiatry

From Philadelphia came Benjamin Rush (1745-1813), whose silhouette was destined to appear on the seal of the American Psychiatric Association, a man whose broad training and many interests rendered him particularly valuable as a co-ordinator of the mental and the physical. He occupied the first chair in chemistry in the United States, but like every alert and versatile mind at the time, he soon branched out and wrote disquisitions on the influence of physical causes upon the moral faculty, on the relations of tastes and aliments, on the state of body and mind in old age, and on the necessity on the part of the ordinary practitioner of injecting himself into the patient's state of mind.

Although a strong believer, Rush was nevertheless inclined to favor physical theories. Thus he thought that "all the operations in the mind are the effects of motions previously excited in the brain and every thought and idea appears to depend upon a motion peculiar to itself." He just misses stumbling on the theory of nerve impulses, and proceeds to tell us that in a sound state of mind these motions are regular and uniform. More physical still is his etiological account of insanity as an arterial disease. This may be true in the case of senile dementia, but what about the many other psychoses? As a chemist, he might have followed a more modern line of reasoning but, apparently, he was no investigator. A man of many convictions which he championed with might and main, his influence stems perhaps more from his practical idealism and his humanitarian efforts than from his actual achievements as a scientist. His preoccupation with bleeding and purging as the panacea for all disease is sufficient evidence of the low state of medical science, nearly two hundred years ago.

THE BEGINNING OF PSYCHOSOMATIC MEDICINE

It is always difficult to state just when a new conception or movement had its inception. Ideas never come into the world full-blown but germinate and grow gradually.

Who would expect a succinct treatise on psychosomatics from the pen of a poet? And yet 180 years ago, the great Friedrich Schiller, poet, dramatist, and historian, in his dissertation written as a candidate for the medical degree at the age of twenty, sketches the relation between mind and body in a remarkably modern vein. "Man is not soul or body," he sets forth. "He is these two substances inmostly united." With an array of apt illustrations, he argues his point effectively. "Sailors drifting about on the ocean and prostrated by the want of bread and water practically recover their health and strength at the sound of 'land' shouted from the masthead." He dilates on apparent exceptions which in reality are only indications of the same law, somewhat askew. Thus an onset of rage may "terminate the most obstinate constipation" or fright relieve "old pains in the limbs or incurable paralysis."

Had Goethe's boon companion stuck to medicine, instead of abandoning it for literature, we might have had an elaboration of the psychosomatic point of view on a textbook scale; for he had a scientifically observant mind. Neglected by both the literary and medical men, Schiller's contribution to medical psychology is scarcely known.

The Founder of Psychosomatic Medicine

It was Ernst von Feuchtersleben (1806-1849), born the year after Schiller's death, who may be spoken of as the founder of psychosomatic medicine as a systematic discipline; for in his *Lehrbuch der ärztlichen Seelenkunde,* published in Vienna in 1845, he gave articulate expression to the principle that man is a psychophysical totality. If he appeared to stress the psychological phase, it is because he was interested in the therapeutic end; and his method of "secondary education" was not unlike Morton Prince's "re-education" technique some 150 years later.

Feuchtersleben held a position of prominence as Dean of the Medical School at the University of Vienna, but dying at the age of forty-three, he was soon forgotten, as other pioneers came on the scene with more searching equipment, until with the rise of the psychosomatic trend, his name was revived.

Griesinger—The First Genuine Psychiatrist

Up to about the middle of the nineteenth century, one could hardly speak of psychiatry as a specialty in the sense of a body of scientific data applicable on a universal scale. There were mental hospitals, clinical surveys, and textbooks, cluttered with nomenclatures which varied from country to country and from decade to decade, and liberally overlaid with so-called histories of patients that were purely descriptive.

Noted medical men in England commanded respect on the Continent. France, because of its progressiveness and variety of abnormal specimens, was the cynosure of the world's alienists. In Germany, the physical and natural sciences prospered, and great names were beginning to loom on the experimental horizon. But when we consider that Heinroth's sermonizing textbook was in use when Griesinger was a student, we shall better understand why the latter was head and shoulders above his predecessor, and why he has been accorded the designation "First Genuine Psychiatrist."

Wilhelm Griesinger (1817-1868) belongs to the titans of medical psychology. He possessed all the necessary endowments for rising to pre-eminence—a precocious interest in the medical sciences rather than in medicine itself, an assimilative mind which could synthesize a conglomeration of facts, a judicious faculty which could discard the speculative and spot what is likely, a freedom from traditional views which enabled him to forge out on his own, and, last but not least, a prodigious capacity for work as well as a practical capacity for obtaining facilities for research. His dignified bearing and success as a lecturer helped his cause, while the journals he founded served to extend his influence beyond Germany.

After receiving his medical degree at the University of Tübingen at the age of twenty-one, he spent a year in Paris and upon his return to Germany, interned for two years, with an eye to engaging in psychiatric work. But he first obtained a thorough grounding in physiology, which had already become an experimental science, thanks to the genius of Johannes Müller.

While still in his twenties, he edited a physiological periodical and published his standard work, *Pathologie und Therapie der Psychischen Krankheiten* (1845), which, in a subsequent edition, was translated into French and English. He was probably the first to treat the psychotic and the neurotic as two separate classifications, at least for clinical purposes. The title of the journal he founded, *Archiv für Psychiatrie und Nervenkrankheiten,* tells the story, but more indicative is the condition he stipulated, on accepting a call to Berlin, that he be given a clinic for the neurotic alongside that for the deranged. His clinical demonstrations were part of the instruction at the Medical School.

According to Zilboorg, Griesinger was a somatologist, pure and simple. Mental diseases were somatic disease, he proclaimed—specifically, diseases of the brain. If we examine Griesinger's textbook, we shall find that the author is not quite so one-sided as Zilboorg interprets him. It is true that Griesinger remarks: "Nothing is more false, nothing is more opposed to everyday observation than any attempt to transpose the nature of the mental diseases into the territory of morality." But practically a whole chapter is devoted to the "I" (*ichheit*), which he takes to be an abstraction containing traces of all former separate sensations, thoughts, and desires, bundled together. Indeed, much of Chapter III could fit into a philosophical text, and some of it reminds us of James's chapter on the self. He may even be considered a forerunner of presentday *ego* psychology, in the dynamic sphere.

The Griesinger textbook is impressive because of the authority behind his statements. Unlike the French texts, there is an aloofness, an impersonal and slightly abstract treatment of the material. The style is more English than German, by no means complicated in its sentence structure; and the careful qualification of statements also savors of English scientific writing.

It is, however, Teutonic in its comprehensiveness, its erudition, and its systematic arrangement. The copious illustrations, most of them culled from foreign periodicals, largely French, are crisp and apt. In other words, one cannot read the book without the feeling that it is the product of a master. He is direct and specific. Yet, there is still a trace of cobweb left in the tidied upper story. Even he thinks that at the acute stage bloodletting "if specially indicated, can have the best results." It is somewhat surprising, too, that he links some cases of insanity with masturbation —certainly a hangover from the older school.

Griesinger's experimental work was instrumental in his favoring the organic etiology of mental disease, but his flashes of intuition in regard to dynamic interpretations reveal another side of his thinking. He sees, for example, in incendiarism the relief through an outward act, no matter how destructive, of the profound discord which the perpetrator has been experiencing.

Yet with all his immense knowledge of physiology and fundamental grasp of pathology, he could not actually prove the connection of organic disease and mental disorder, except where there was a definite degeneration of brain tissue, permitting no doubt, as in general paresis or senile dementia (though he did not associate general paresis with syphilis, as was later established). He makes use of such qualifiers as "probably," "sometimes," "here may exist," "not uncommon," etc. when he wishes to point out the organic causes of insanity. That there may be somatic concomitants of mental disturbances does not clinch the issue. Thus he believes that anemia can cause insanity, or that morbid conditions of genital organs have an important influence in this regard. Apparently Griesinger is a better critic of others' views than of his own.

On the other hand, when he expatiates on the behavior of patients and the evaluation of their motives, he seems to be without a peer until the advent of psychoanalysis. His views on suicide, as contrasted with those of the French alienists, are eminently modern.

Griesinger's greatest service was in the building of clinics and in the detailed examination, from all angles, of both mild and serious cases of mental disorder. There is much in his textbook of over a century ago which can be read with profit even today. Had he been less of a pathologist, he might have reached greater heights as a psychiatrist. Where he was unencumbered by his preoccupation with physical causes, he delivered himself of rare insights, and had he not died in middle age, he might have given us the system of classification later contributed by Kraepelin.

Patron Saint of the Insane

We now turn to an American woman who singlehandedly did more for the insane than any psychiatrist.

Born in 1802, Dorothea Lynde Dix was treated so harshly by her parents that at the age of ten she left home. At fourteen, she began teaching school at Worcester, and despite her frail constitution, with a touch of tuberculosis, she managed to win the respect of class after class of pupils, writing a series of books largely for adolescents and for family reading. Because of her worsening state of health, she was obliged to give up her regular schedule, and took the assignment of instructing a class of women prisoners, on Sundays. Her first glimpse of prison life led her to investigate conditions at almshouses, insane asylums, and jails—and she was horrified at what she saw. Still in her thirties and in delicate health, she undertook a herculean task and became the "patron saint of the insane," as she was known in later life.

Within three years she visited eighteen state prisons and three hundred jails, five hundred almshouses, hospitals, and houses of refuge, traveling ten thousand miles in all kinds of weather and on roads which were scarcely viable. She did this on her own funds, having come into a modest patrimony. Her mission seemed to many a forlorn cause, but she succeeded in inspiring influential people with her zeal and humanity; and her memorandum to Congress, in which she describes the insane she found in closets, cellars, cages, pens, naked and chained, beaten and flogged, bore fruit. Replacing the eight asylums which this country had in 1840, many modern hospitals for the insane were built and administered by men trained for the job. Millions of dollars were appropriated by some twenty states, which responded to her call.

During the Civil War, she became chief of the hospital nurses, and later her restless spirit took her to Canada, England and Scotland, where she met with equal success. Queen Victoria, thanks to Dorothea Dix's pleading, asked for a royal commission to investigate insane asylums in Scotland. She was also instrumental in founding a new hospital in Rome.

At an advanced age, she heard of the dangerous shores of Sable Island in Newfoundland, and at once she visited that remote region, moving heaven and earth until life-saving boats were supplied. The following week, a large vessel landed with 168 passengers, who might have lost their lives had it not been for the provision of the boats.

Dorothea Dix died in 1887, at the age of eighty-five. A richly carved monument was erected in her honor. In her singleness of purpose and resolution she reminds us of Florence Nightingale, but she appears to have been more judicious in the selection of her means and less temperamental in her dealings with those in high places.

Morel

The dynasty which began with Pinel, at the Salpêtrière, found in Benedict A. Morel (1809-1873), who was for a time an assistant and secretary to Falret, a psychopathologist comparing favorably with any of his predecessors, at least in point of research.

Born in Germany, and educated in France, he possessed the happy combination of long-nervedness and patience, which is often lacking in the French savant, and the intuitive flashes for which French intellectuals are so noted.

His experience as physician-in-chief, first at the Mareville Asylum and later at an asylum in Rouen, prepared him for the series of investigations associated with his name. For it was not as an administrator, but as an expert on insanity that he won recognition, to the extent that he was called to Munich to offer his opinion on the mental status of a nobleman charged with murder. Thanks to his testimony, the accused was not executed. The man's condition, which at the time was not manifest, soon developed into a full-blown psychosis.

One of the remarkable incidents in his life was his correct prognosis of the later mad Ludwig of Bavaria in the presence of his royal father, who was showing him off to his visitor—an audacious utterance on the part of the scientist.

Morel was perhaps the first to write (in conjunction with Lasèque) a complete survey of psychiatry in half a dozen European countries and the United States. His next large work was *Etudes Médico-psychologiques sur l'aliénation Mentale*. Here he develops the sociological aspects of mental disease, sometimes wavering between the purely psychological, the somatic, and the environmental stress. It was Morel who first described the symptoms of schizophrenia, to which he gave the name of *Démence précoce*, i.e., dementia praecox. His treatise on degeneration alone would secure him a niche in the history of psychiatry. In this book, we already have the basis of the later theory of Lombroso.

As Morel advanced in age, he focused attention on the factors responsible for mental disorders. In his *Traité des Maladies Mentales* (1860) he elaborates on the premise of degeneration, which could be a hereditary matter or due to the influence of various toxins or biological deficiencies. By examining the periphery instead of dwelling on behavior symptoms and classifications, he broadened the scope of the field. His extension of the legal phases of insanity added to his laurels, but since his young contemporary, Magnan, was taking up the same problems with greater specialization, and Charcot subsequently gave a new direction to that branch of medicine, Morel's star began to wane, so that he is scarcely mentioned in present-day textbooks.

BERNHARD A. GUDDEN (1824-1886)
Victim of Royal Maniac

If Bernhard Gudden had not been one of the greatest psychiatrists of the day, he might have lived to a ripe old age, but as fate would have it, he was the victim of a royal maniac.

A dynamic personality, an able administrator, an organizer whose energetic enterprises advanced the cause of his art and science, the editor of the leading psychiatric journal in Germany, he was the natural choice of King Ludwig II of Bavaria for his personal physician. Gudden was just the man to deal with a mad king. He was mature and able to get along with all sorts of people. His build, self-confidence and devotion to his patients and concern for the mentally ill in general were all qualifications that rendered him just the man in whose hands could be intrusted the ruler, whose aberrations were a great trial to the populace of Bavaria.

Dutifully Gudden steered the royal psychotic through the straits of despair, but the crafty monarch had conceived a plan to put an end to his misery. One fine day Ludwig proposed to go sailing, taking his physician along. Apparently the King made an attempt to commit suicide by drowning, which Gudden tried to avert, but although himself robust, he could not cope with the manic strength of his patient, and both patient and physician went down struggling.

Gudden's early work comprised experiments on eye movement and the crossing of nerve fiber in the optical chiasma, as well as on parasites in connection with scabies.

Magnan

Valentine J.-J. Magnan (1835-1916) might be considered a member of the same French dynasty, since he began his career at Bicêtre, where Pinel made his start, and like Morel, caine under the tutelage of Falret.

Magnan was an experimenter, in the modern sense, and a clinician who was interested in advancing our knowledge of the causative factors in mental disease. He was primarily a laboratory man, but he did not rest content with theoretical results, and became an advocate of reform. He threw overboard restraints except on extraordinary occasions and was the first to study alcoholism in a scientific manner. It was largely through his researches that the relationship of tabes to general paresis was established, and his magisterial work on the effects of various liquors, especially absinthe, which in his day was the most popular drink, as well as narcotics, proved of the greatest value in coping with the deteriorating situation after the French defeat in the Franco-Prussian War.

Thanks to his researches on convulsions, delirium, etc., a number of the older ideas had to be modified; and the difference between organic and non-organic mental disease began to appear less misty. Like Morel, Magnan was convinced that heredity played the major part in insanity.

Among the first to introduce clinical demonstrations in his courses, he was taken to task by the press, who decried the practice unethical, branding it as an injustice toward the insane. For a period of two years, the course was suspended by the government.

Magnan seems to have been the first to describe sexual perversions and defects of the genital organs with illustrations. His *Recherches sur la Dégenera-*

tion takes up such subjects as the criminally insane, onomatomania (i.e., the compulsion to repeat a certain word or name or being so affected by it as to dread it), and paranoia.

His *Leçons Cliniques sur les Maladies Mentales* constituted his course of lectures and was brought out by two of his former students, and translated into German by Paul Möbius.

Charcot and His Magic Wand

In Jean-Martin Charcot (1825-1893), French psychiatry reached a new high; and La Salpêtrière through him became known throughout Europe as the happy hunting-ground for young physicians who were seeking variegated experience in the psychiatric field. Its reputation had grown since the time of Pinel, but it was Charcot's aura which lent it a special luster.

Charcot, the son of an humble coach-maker, made his début in medicine with a dissertation on rheumatism. In 1850, he became a laureate of the hospitals, and in 1852, a laureate of the medical faculty. Many branches of medicine claimed his attention, diseases of the vascular system, lungs, liver and kidneys, skin, Basedow's disease, and even cancer. He had had a thorough grounding in physiology, which later formed the basis of his laboratory work, in collaboration with his assistants, later incorporated in *Leçons sur les Maladies sur le Système Nerveux*, 1887-1888.

In 1866, he took charge of the service of La Salpêtrière, and having married the widowed daughter of a Maecenas, his influence and effectualness were increased through his affluence and extra-professional position. It was his dominant personality, however, that counted most. There was something theatrical in his bearing. A man of striking appearance, decisive movements, and great self-assurance, he was admired and respected by his subordinates and associates. He always knew what he wanted, and possessed the means of securing it.

He made La Salpêtrière glamorous by equipping the institution with adequate laboratories, art studios and offices, and clinics for physiotherapy, electrotherapy, and ophthalmology. His success as a lecturer was enormous. In 1872, he was elected to the French Academy of Medicine. At first, his title was Professor of Pathological Anatomy, but before long, he founded the clinical chair for nervous diseases, and was its first incumbent. Interested in art, he co-authored *Les Démoniques dans l'Art* and *Les Difformes et les Malades dans l'Art.*

It may be mentioned that his son Jean-Baptiste, who also set out on a medical career, gained glory subsequently as an explorer whose adventures in the Antarctic and Arctic regions gave the world most valuable scientific data. An intrepid navigator of his ship *Pourquoi-Pas,* after the most perilous encounters with the elements, he met death in an explosion just as he was leaving a port in Iceland. In French reference works he is accorded almost twice as much space as his celebrated father, for whom, incidentally, he named a piece of territory he discovered in the Antarctic.

Whether or not Charcot was convinced that all mental disease is due to organic causes is not easy to judge. Brain physiology, or neurology, promised so much during the whole century that a scientist could not neglect such researches, even if they offered nothing conclusive; and it can scarcely be said that Charcot's two volumes proved any more than those of his French or German predecessors.

It was in another sphere that Charcot made his mark. Focusing on the milder abnormalities, like hysteria, he proceeded to enlighten the thousands of students who sat at his feet with spectacular clinical displays. During that period there seems to have been a recrudescence of hysteria reminiscent of the demonism of the late Renaissance, except that the susceptible were no longer burnt as witches or tortured to wrest confessions from them.

Charcot paraded an interminable array of hysterics, whom he would hypnotize, and who, he thought, fell into three successive stages of sleep—lethargy, catalepsy, and somnambulism—a supposition which was not generally accepted, for it was difficult to find a line of demarcation between the lighter and deeper forms of the trance.

Perhaps the chief service of Charcot was in pointing the way toward a psychogenic conception of the neuroses. Since hysteria belonged to the milder mental disorders; and since nothing could be found in the musculature to warrant spells of paralysis or of anaesthesia, such conditions must be induced by self-imposed ideas; and their temporary nature seemed to confirm such a surmise.

There was a temptation on the part of Charcot to associate hysteria with some uterine condition, more specifically the ovaries; and Freud tells us that while he was a student at Salpêtrière, Charcot, in the course of describing a certain case, raised himself on his toes and confidentially remarked, "*Mais, toujours c'est la chose génitale, toujours.*" Freud thought it strange that his chief could recognize the fact without making it part of his system. It was well, perhaps, that Charcot did not follow up his clue; or the wholesale ovariotomies and hysterectomies of our time might have started some eighty years ago.

Perhaps it was the concomitance of convulsions with some of the hysterias that caused him to link hysteria with epilepsy; and in accordance with the division of epilepsy into *petit mal* and *gros mal,* he spoke of minor and major hysteria, which may have belonged nosologically to two different orders of disease.

Another of his slips was his view that the various

hypnotic phenomena are fundamentally associated with hysteria; in other words, that they might constitute a diagnostic clue. This is reminiscent of the attitude of the inquisitors, who were certain that if a woman could feel no pain when pricked by a pin, she must be possessed by the Devil. We shall see how Bernheim was closer to the truth about the nature of hypnotism, which Charcot fancied to have some magnetic influence, from which the normal person was protected. In this respect, he differed from Mesmer, who had been discredited by the Académie des Sciences more than sixty years earlier.

Charcot's mantle fell upon Janet, who broke with the tradition of searching for the physiological causes of mental disorders. The time was ripe for a return to the psychological conception; and Freud was beginning to explore not so much the inferno as the purgatory of human ills—both Janet and Freud keeping closer to the ubiquitous neurotic than to that greater deviant, the psychotic.

BERNHEIM AND THE WORLD OF SUGGESTION

Like other leaders in their particular field, Charcot had his opposite number. It was Hippolyte M. Bernheim (1840-1919), a Jewish physician who was in charge of the Nancy Asylum and taught at the University. It is true that Bernheim did not cut as wide a swath as did Charcot. He did not attract physicians from all parts of the world to witness his awesome demonstrations of hysteric women falling into deep trances. But Bernheim's rival views on hysteria and hypnotism stood the test of time as against those of the celebrated Charcot. Furthermore, the man who came under his influence and even translated his book on suggestion and hypnotism into German, with a lengthy preface of his own, was Sigmund Freud, then a clinic "explorer."

Bernheim, whose family came from Alsace, which has furnished France with many of her luminaries, had worked along the borderline of the mental and the physical. He had published a little book on aphasia and one on typhus, and was hardly more than a general practitioner, when he made the acquaintance of Ambroise A. Liébeault (1823-1904), who had become interested in hypnotism after listening to a report of Braid's work before the French Académie des Sciences. James Braid (1795-1860), a Manchester physician, was the man who stole the thunder of mesmerism and called it "hypnotism," the art of putting people to sleep, at the same time exposing the hoax of the *baquet* and the fallacy of animal magnetism which Mesmer and his followers were, as he thought, palming off on the credulous.

Braid was the creative type, a writer and experimenter, and with the ambition to push his ideas. Liébeault, on the other hand, was more like the country doctor, who had his own methods and was willing to adopt new ideas and techniques, but because of his non-aggressive personality, his conservative colleagues only poked fun at him.

In 1883, when Bernheim was forty-three, he sent a patient suffering from sciatica to Liébeault and was amazed to find the patient cured. At once, he, the rising scientist, became the exponent of Liébeault's method.

While it was true that Bernheim had been put on the right track by Liébeault, yet without Bernheim's theoretical groundwork of the method he employed, Liébeault's name would now be unknown.

Hypnotism as a phenomenon had been known for ages, through an evolution of names and stages, yet the whole field was pervaded by a heavy mist.

The controversy between Charcot and Bernheim came to be known as the difference between the Paris (or La Salpêtrière) and Nancy schools. Bernheim's view, which represents hypnotism as merely an exaggerated form of suggestion and different only in degrees from the phenomena of normal mental life, won out against the complicated, almost mystical, doctrine of Charcot. In criticism of Charcot, Bernheim employs a *reductio ad absurdum* argument when he points out that were hypnotism a function only of the hysterical whose nerves are wrought up, since we all have nerves and tend to be excited and can be hypnotized, then we should all be classed as hysterics. Students of psychology and psychopathology nowadays take Bernheim's conclusions for granted, oblivious of the rough path that the Nancy leader had to travel. With what skepticism Bernheim's rational views were received may be seen from the comment in *La Grande Encyclopédie* to the effect that, although his researches are of the greatest interest, they need confirmation.

Bernheim, who thought that all persons who believed they could be hypnotized were susceptible, as against Charcot, who declared hypnotism *a function of the abnormal only,* had to contend with many opponents. Dubois, for instance, criticized him on the ground that he claimed to cure all mental ills through suggestion, whereas Dubois believed that only in some of the psychoneuroses—nervous aphonia, functional paralysis, nervous vomiting, or the psychic anesthesias and the like—is suggestion applicable; while in the neurasthenias and psychasthenias, which are to him of toxic origin, involving constitutional factors, suggestion is of no more avail than in the psychoses.

Defending himself against the strictures of Dubois, Bernheim institutes an important distinction between *credivity,* which he regards as the normal capacity for belief, even where there is no demonstration before our eyes, and credulity, which is *excessive* credivity.[32] Yet in the latter case, the cerebral cells which accept the idea do not implement the nerves, as in the case of credivity, to *realize* it. In credivity, ideodynamic action does follow.

In simple terms, suggestion consists of causing certain brain paths to become clear while others are closed. It is a physiological process induced by the suggester.

About thirty years ago, it will be recalled, a dapper Nancy druggist caused a stir in the world with a new form of therapy, namely, autosuggestion. He was Emile Coué, whose little refrain,

Every day, in every way
I am getting better and better,

became the rage of the stray as well as of the gay; and the newspaper guild—columnist, cartoonist, and editorialist—had the time of their life with the new formula. Coué insisted that the imagination was stronger than the will, and all you had to do was imagine that you were getting better and better, and the cure was sure-fire. Bernheim's technique was quite different.

In order to understand the halo which surrounded Bernheim in the late nineties, it is necessary to read the account of the Nancy School by van Renterghem in the *Zeitschrift für Hypnotismus* (1896, Vol. V), himself a leading physician, won over to the new psychotherapeutic method.

> One must needs have seen him operate in his service in order to understand how he had attained such remarkable success.
>
> He is small in stature. His eyes are blue and mild and yet penetrating. He has a gentle but persuasive voice. As I was accompanying him through his service at the *hôpital civil,* during his call there, he led me from bed to bed, explaining each of the cases and giving proof of his mastery in the art of diagnosis.

In *Le Magnétisme Animal* (1889), Delboeuf, one of the leading French scientists, devotes a number of pages to a vivid description of Bernheim's technique. The conversation between physician and patient is recorded verbatim. Sufferers too ignorant to understand what is expected of them, or too incredulous to take the instructions seriously, are put to sleep by the determined physician, and awaken to find themselves, if not entirely cured, at least very much improved:

> "Let's see. Where does it hurt you?"
> "In the head."

"Your headache will disappear: it's gone, it's over! You feel no more pain."

"No."

"Are you asleep?"

"I don't think so."

"You are asleep! You'll not remember anything on awakening. You don't feel anything." (He is pricked) "When you awake you'll drink half a glass of water."

In less time than it takes to write this, Delboeuf declares, the man was sound asleep, and it was evident that the patient was no longer suffering.

From several eminent neurologists, who enjoyed the opportunity of witnessing the memorable clinical treatments by the Nancy master, I have heard similar comments on his prowess in the clinic. His walking down the corridor and putting the patients to sleep by the magic spell of his "*dormez, dormez, dormez*" has remained a vivid memory with many a practitioner of yesteryear who was fortunate to witness his demonstrations.

Maudsley, the Clinician-Theorist

The most outstanding psychiatrist in the British Isles, next to Tuke, was Henry Maudsley (1835-1918), who looked as if he might have been a sibling of Charles Darwin, except that he wore a more patriarchal beard and a decidedly prophetic air, pensive and wistful.

Educated at the University of London, where years later, he served as a professor of medical jurisprudence, he was nurtured upon the pioneer works of Darwin, Tyndall, Huxley, and Spencer, during the heyday of evolutionary thought. Since Maudsley was a child of his era, we might well surmise that his philosophy would brook no tinge of metaphysics.

Like his predecessors of the previous century, he believed in the empirical method and would have no truck with anything which was intangible. That did not prevent him from theorizing, but always in a physicalistic vein. As with Huxley, in his system consciousness was only an epiphenomenon, and although he made many references to the "unconscious" it certainly is not the unconscious of Freud, but rather the cerebration of nerve impulses. It was indeed because of frequent confusion that the term "subconscious" was used in many English books to designate Freud's concept.

Actually it was the physiologist W. B. Carpenter who, in 1852, introduced the term "unconscious cerebration," [33] which must have been adopted by the growing Maudsley. Although Carpenter was an older contemporary, both seem to represent one concern on the issue of body and mind, and their point of view has permeated the curriculum even of high schools both in England and the United States, as may be seen from the examination paper in Thayer Academy, in 1894, which I found in the library of William James about thirty-five years ago.

Even Münsterberg, who did not, by any means, scout philosophy, denied the existence of "the subconscious," and made the pronunciamento that a process was either conscious or unconscious, and attributed the unconscious solving of problems to physiological cerebration.

Medical men in pre-Freudian days were prone to accept this conclusion as self-evident and the opposite view as mystical. Carpenter and Maudsley were names frequently seen in textbooks and heard at lectures and in seminars some fifty years ago.

In keeping with the philosophy of Herbert Spencer and the evolutionists in general, Maudsley thought in terms of adaptation. Thus, to him, "Insanity marks a failure in organic adaptation to external nature;

it is the result and evidence of a discord between the man and his surroundings: he cannot bend circumstances to himself nor accommodate himself to circumstances."[34] This forms the original basis of the social worker's platform, adopted especially in the United States. The sociological bias may be inferred from the following passage in his *Physiology and Pathology of the Mind:*

> The organ of the mind unconsciously appropriates through the inlets of the senses the influence of its surroundings. . . . An individual may consciously arrange the circumstances in which he will live, but cannot prevent the conscious assimilation of their influence, and the corresponding modification of his character; not only slight habits of movements are thus acquired but habits of thought and feeling are imperceptibly organized; so that an acquired nature may ultimately govern one who is not at all conscious that he has changed.

Paradoxically, Maudsley, like Freud, is of the opinion that all this physiological going-on takes place in the mind. In other words, the mind is to him coextensive on a parallel basis with the brain, while consciousness is not.

Against the backdrop of evolution and unconscious cerebration, as well as British traditional empiricism, Maudsley's theory of mental disease is in line with the somatic conception that some brain twist or lesion is responsible for the disorder.

His experience as a medical superintendent of the Manchester Royal Lunatic Asylum and as physician in the West London Hospital was well utilized in the writing of his major works: *The Physiology and Pathology of Mind* and *Organic to Human; Psychological and Sociological* (1917). His humanitarian traits found expression in his generous gift of thirty thousand pounds (almost $150,000 and equivalent to nearly half a million dollars today) to erect a psychiatric hospital in London. This hospital, named for him, is one of the best-conducted institutions in the United Kingdom.

J. L. A. KOCH (1841-1908)
The Explorer of Psychopathic Inferiority

While some of the French alienists had already dwelt on the so-called "psychopathic inferiorities," describing many of them in detail, Koch, in German fashion, systemized them, and indicated definite stages, such as (a) the *dispositional,* where only a tendency can be spotted; (b) the *stigmatic;* and (c) the *degenerative.* He speaks of two different groups, the innate and the acquired. As to the former, he believed, with most of his colleagues, that the cause was a diseased condition of the brain.

In *Die abnormen Charaktere* (1900) he attempts to demarcate the line between normality and abnormality, and tells us that "by far the majority of those who suffer from psychopathic inferiority are not less adequate than the average person. . . . Many of those psychopathically inferior tower above other people, exhibit great talent, fine feelings, and are energetic in action, possess noble characters, and are scholars, prominent men."

The chief symptoms of such inferiorities Koch had already described in his earlier textbook, *Leitfaden der Psychiatrie* (1888), but it is in his chief work, *Die psychopathischen Minderwertigkeiten* (1891-1893), that he relieves himself of some provocative paradoxes. For example: "Many *minderwertige* [inferiors] are *mehr werth* [more worthy] in their psychic life than many others who are perfectly sound." Not even Freud has surpassed some of the interpretations of neurotic behavior we find in Koch, who nevertheless cautions us against finding psychopathic inferiorities everywhere. "They are most unusually prevalent, more so than is supposed, but they do not exist everywhere."

Ziehen and Kraepelin mention him approvingly in their respective textbooks, but it is not given to the Kochs, with their personal handicaps, to cut a figure among their colleagues. It is evident that he was not aggressive enough.

Möbius—The Originator of Pathography

One of the most fertile-minded writers in the field was P. J. Möbius (1853-1907). His name carries little weight at present, yet he may be regarded as the creator of the branch of psychiatry to which the name of pathography was given.

Psychoanalysis has exploited this area with great avidity, but it was Möbius who opened it up through his searching examination of the behavior of famous men, who were often thought of as practically without faults, their quirks discounted as wrinkles that could be dismissed in the light of their circumstances.

It redounds to the credit of Möbius, the son of a well-known mathematician, that he treated many of the world's geniuses as in some respect psychopathic. He had no difficulty, of course, proving the paranoid trait in Jean Jacques Rousseau, but to make Goethe an abnormal required some courage. Yet in the compass of two volumes, he relates so many instances of Goethe's non-rational behavior and brings to the fore so many changes of his mood that one is inclined to conclude that the greatest genius Germany produced was what we would today call a mild manic-depressive.

The lives of Schopenhauer and of Nietzsche, particularly the latter, gave him little trouble, for Nietzsche spent his last days in an insane asylum, but to trace the development of the psychosis in Nietzsche's normal life took a brilliant mind to undertake and carry out.

Every monograph which came from the pen of Möbius teemed with pregnant thoughts, even if we are not disposed to accept them all. He could champion unpopular causes, as when he agreed to some extent with Gall the phrenologist; and in a book on mathematical endowment, argued on the basis of cranial conformations in mathematicians that there is a particular region at the forefront of the brain which is the organ of this endowment.[35] Moreover, he thought there were types of mathematicians—the algebraists and the geometricians each requiring a different kind of imagery—also that the French excelled in the one while the Germans were more proficient in the other.

Kraepelin, in his textbook,[36] credits him with the origination of the two types of etiology in mental disease: exogenous, that is, those disorders which are caused by outside factors; and endogeneous, those which stem from congenital or constitutional defects.

We thus see that there were tangential points between Möbius and the later Lombroso school (Max Nordau), the psychoanalysts, looking for kinks in every individual, and the typologists. His work on the mental inferiority of women because of physiological causes evoked a good deal of criticism from various quarters.

Kraepelin—The Systematizer

German psychiatry had been making strides since Heinroth, and Griesinger particularly had rescued it from the doldrums of verbiage and pedantic nomenclature, but Emil Kraepelin (1855-1926) was the man who brought it to its pinnacle. He seems to have been the epitome of all who preceded him, and may be considered as the follower of Griesinger, insofar as he, too, believed in the somatic source of all mental disease. Revising and enlarging his *Psychiatrie—ein Lehrbuch,* which he first published at the age of twenty-eight, Kraepelin made out of it a work of four hefty volumes (eighth edition) comprising nearly 2,500 pages, in which every nook and cranny of psychiatry was examined and its contents brought to light.

Kraepelin was able to accomplish more than Griesinger, not only because he lived twenty years longer, but because he was more the researcher, and less the administrator. He was a glutton for work, and it is not just a coincidence that the journal he founded in 1897, and which died with him, was called *Psychologische Arbeiten.* Work was his gospel, and although he did not preach it, as did Carlyle, he certainly treated it as a sort of religion.

Contribution to Psychology

There was one other respect in which Kraepelin had the advantage over Griesinger. He was schooled in experimental psychology, and was one of the first students to enroll in the first psychological laboratory. Wundt's influence was gratefully acknowledged in a little book which he dedicated to the master. In this compact survey, he presented the results of his experiments to show the effects of certain drugs on a number of mental processes. One senses a note of hopefulness rather than the expression of satisfaction in the concluding paragraph:

> At the beginning of experimental psychological studies, everything appears to be so easily without order, fortuitous, contradictory; we see here, however, that the conformity of law finally does emerge, that the impressions of subjective experience must finally lead to tangible scientific

formulation even in the sphere of individual psychology. The task is difficult and thorny, no doubt, but insoluble it does not appear to me.

General psychology is beholden to Kraepelin in no small measure; for his laboratory was organized as no other in this field, with specific problems assigned to graduate students and assistants. There were investigations on the depth of sleep, ergographical studies, experiments on expectation, surprise, and disappointment. Aschaffenburg's noted experiments on association, which Jung later adapted to psychoneurotic cases, were conducted in Kraepelin's laboratory; and here the British psychologist, Rivers, worked on fatigue and recovery. Kraepelin was the first to study the effect of work pauses on mental accomplishment, and the effect of tea, alcohol, bromides, formaldehyde, and ether on mental processes.

His standards were rigid. Whether he could satisfy present-day statistical requirements is doubtful, but his computations were painstakingly charted, and his methodology was superior to that of the French and Belgian investigators, like Morel and Magnan, who were tackling similar problems.

His chief contribution was the work curve, establishing the process at every stage. W. Weygandt, who wrote an elaborate obituary in *Psychologische Arbeiten,* reveals that Kraepelin had hoped to receive the Nobel award for his labors on the work curve. A naïve expectation, perhaps, but it shows how much weight he placed on those extensive researches.

Contribution to Psychiatry

In psychiatry, Kraepelin has been hailed as the man who, once and for all, brought system into the classification of psychoses. Whether he introduced revolutionary ideas into the whole field is doubtful. Even the terms *dementia praecox* and *manic-depres-*

sive were not entirely new. Morel, in 1860, had already used the term *démence précoce*, and in 1684, Théophile Bonet (1620-1689) had used the term *folie maniaco-mélancolique*. The term *folie circulaire* was introduced by Esquirol's successor, Falret, so that the nature of this disease was known long before Kraepelin. It remained for him to consolidate the knowledge and concatenate the *disjecta membra* found in the various treatises.

If his predecessors, especially the French clinicians, may be said to have used a magnifying glass in their observations, then Kraepelin may be said to have examined details with a strong microscope. Abreast of all the psychological and psychopathological literature of the day, he was able to relate one set of minutiae to another, until the jigsaw puzzle made sense.

For the first time, the picture of dementia praecox embraced all types of cases. In his classification, the various catatonic reactions, hebephrenia, and mixed or borderline types are, at long last, fully described and illustrated. The same is true of the other large class of diseases—the manic-depressives, which are also pinpointed in the most orderly fashion. More aloof from the patient than, say, Pinel or Esquirol, Kraepelin saw motives in a different light. The contradictions themselves, to Kraepelin, followed a regular course.

Kraepelin thought that while manic-depressive cases could recover, schizophrenia was far more serious because the tendency toward deterioration was progressive. If someone diagnosed as schizophrenic did get well, the assumption must be either that the case had not been properly diagnosed in the first place, or else that the recuperant would experience a relapse. Prognosis, then, in Kraepelin's system became the condition or even the criterion for diagnosis—and that, too, on a premise which begs the question. It was because of Kraepelin's supposition that schizophrenia was incurable that so little was done in most institutions to find better treatment than the hospital routine. For many of these patients, the inscription to Dante's inferno could have been borrowed as a sign at the entrance of the ward. There was more faith in the Italian and French clinicians.

Kraepelin's road to success was not an easy one. His recognition as the arbiter in psychiatric issues came late in life and grew after his death. Many clinicians considered him a plodder who spent a great deal of time and energy obtaining results which they would be able to gather through their daily observations or infer as a matter of course. He sometimes projected opposing theories which threatened to topple the structure he had erected. These he would take cognizance of in later editions of his textbook. To take one instance: sudden seizures of violence, or paroxysms of laughter, or spells of unaccountable anxiety are, according to Bleuler, explained by the touching off of complexes in the schizophrenic. Kraepelin, on the other hand, attributes them to the loss of balancing and controlling values, which the normal person possesses.[37]

Kraepelin's classification of psychoses has been generally accepted, with some modifications in consequence of cases which do not fit into the original scheme. Much greater hope is now held out for the schizophrenic, especially since experiments with certain drugs like mescaline and lysergic acid have shown that certain of the symptoms can be artificially induced in mild and temporary form. It must not be forgotten, however, that Kraepelin was the most persistent experimenter, decades earlier, in the effect of drugs on the mind.

In one of his many enlightening and entertaining conversations, Morton Prince told the author how, at a dinner given Kraepelin in Boston, the latter turned his glass upside down when it was about to be filled with liquor. Prince criticized the action as lacking in tact, as if he were censuring those who drank alcohol. He also told of Kraepelin's taking the trouble to untie the knot around a parcel, because it was more ethical than to cut it. A matter of ethics or not, it demonstrates Kraepelin's enormous self-discipline.

The man who, as Weygandt tells us, had difficulty entering the medical faculty at the University of Leipzig became one of its resplendent ornaments, a situation reminiscent of the metaphor in *Psalms:* "The stone, rejected by the masons, has become the corner-piece" in the end.

Dubois and the Psychoneuroses

Paul Dubois (1848-1918), one of the most popular names fifty years ago, when Jelliffe and his alter ego, W. A. White, translated his chief work on nervous disorders, is today hardly known even in psychiatric circles. Freud, in his derogatory reference to Jung's conception, implies that Dubois was his inspiration. Although both Jung and Dubois are Swiss, it is not likely that the latter had influenced Jung in any way. The moral aspect in psychotherapy is what links the two.

Dubois was primarily a psychotherapist. Perhaps it was because somatic research did not appeal to him that he centered his attention on what we call the psychoneuroses. The very title of one of his books, "*Die Einbildung als Krankheitsursache*" (*Imagination as Cause of Disease*) shows that he belongs with the French alienists, antedating the more recent trends in para-Freudianism, which stress the rôle of the self and the function of the will in effecting a cure. His once popular *Education of the Self* is not without some value for the neurotic who wants to help himself. Nor is *Les Psychoneuroses et Leur Traitement Moral* (1904) to be brushed aside.

The principle which operates in Dubois's system is moral suasion—an echo of Heinroth's theological psychiatry. Dubois, however, merely sees in the decent life the *sine qua non* of integration. When the individual falters or stumbles, he can straighten himself out, generally with the aid of the practitioner, through re-education. In this we can spot an anticipation of Morton Prince's technique in treating the milder disorders, as well as of the para-Freudian tendencies of the last two decades to lay more emphasis on the ego and its requirements—in other words, the character elements rather than the wholly unconscious mechanisms without reference to the moral values. Nor was Dubois's treatment simply a matter of suggestion, or less still, autosuggestion.

When, therefore, Freud sarcastically asks whether it is necessary to hark back to Dubois by way of Jung, he intimates that both are preachers or prophets rather than scientists. Certainly Dubois was no Kraepelin, nor Charcot, nor Freud, but his experience with patients was extensive, and his treatment was effective, while his books, without pretense of elaborate research, were sound presentations of the lesser mental troubles and contained much wisdom. His conferences with the mentally ill were a species of psychoanalysis, minus the system.

Bleuler's Innovations

Of higher caliber was another Swiss psychiatrist, who may take his place beside the shining lights of the latter half of the nineteenth century. That was Eugen Bleuler (1857-1939), but for whom and his assistant, C. G. Jung, Zürich would have been known for other things than psychiatry.

Bleuler's conspicuous service in the understanding of the most common mental trouble started when he changed the name of dementia praecox to schizophrenia, which he defined as a specific kind of alteration of thought and feeling and relations with the outer world.

He was sympathetic to Freud's doctrines, although

he was far from going the whole hog with psychoanalysis; and its founder was apparently disappointed after rejoicing in so important a sponsorship. His descriptions of the psychotic, unlike the earlier French matter-of-fact protocols, operated in the sphere of the unconscious, in the motivational; and therefore, his mechanisms often converged with those of Freud, from whom he may have gained a broader vision as regards interpretation. In other words, *Bleuler has definitely entered the dynamic area.* Thus we find him encouraging Jung in his association investigations, and it was not Jung who steered Bleuler in the direction of Freud but the other way around. Bleuler came to the conclusion that in the schizophrenic, *the associations tend to loosen and disintegrate.* Often the logical gives way to the verbal; for example, the patient, when asked whether his thoughts are heavy, will miss the metaphoric sense and reply, "Yes, iron is heavy."

Among the mechanisms, conditions, and tendencies which Bleuler finds in the schizophrenic are: (a) condensation; (b) displacement of ideas, as when a symbol is used that is only remotely related to the object; (c) absence of a central idea; (d) gross generalization; (e) unrelated reasoning; and, of course, (e) delusions; and what Bleuler calls dereistic thinking, that is, altogether unrelated to an object—"something thinks" for the patient. Perseveration and the flight of ideas, while not peculiar to schizophrenia, are, despite their disparate categories, to be expected in the same individual. The contradiction is even more pronounced in such mental processes as arithmetic. At one moment, he will not be able to add two numbers, and shortly thereafter, he will extract the cube root of a given number.

When Bleuler substituted the term schizophrenia for dementia praecox, it was because he felt the most characteristic thing about the disease was the split of the personality's unity, so that there appear to be two parallel courses in the mind. The affects especially lose their cohesion, and we have what he calls "parathymia"—not simply an alternation of mood or temper but a kind of contradictory feeling. Again, Bleuler found it necessary to coin the term "ambivalence," which has been adopted in psychoanalysis. The possibility of hating and loving an object or person at the same time, to a logically minded individual, seemed utter nonsense, but the schizophrenic does not move in a logical ambit.

Another term Bleuler is responsible for is "*syntonic,*" which he substituted for the cycloid type. We may wonder at such an elevation of the cycloid, and, by comparison, the demotion of the schizoid; for "syntonic" implies well-balanced, harmonious; but let us remember that, as in Kretschmer's dichotomy, the categories are only biotypes, matrices, out of which, under special circumstances, there emerge pathological conditions. The two biotypes correspond also to Jung's extraverts and introverts. The former is generally thought of as the "regular guy," while the latter is considered a "queer duck," and if the tension becomes unbearable he will turn schizophrenic, with all that this implies prognostically.

The phrase "escape from reality" seems to cover the general picture of the schizophrenic in Bleuler's gallery. The phrase "autistic thinking," as when a psychotic hands someone a piece of toilet paper and maintains it's a check, is Bleuler's coinage.

Bleuler is inclined to the hereditarian conception, but is not committed to the somatic doctrine of mental illness. The only concession he makes is to introduce the potency of hormones as bearing on the development of schizophrenia, but that, again, only as a hypothesis. He does not believe in drugs as direct remedies, and recommends their avoidance, though they may be resorted to as a palliative in emergency cases.

To summarize his large *Lehrbuch der Psychiatrie*

(1916) or his *Naturgeschichte der Seele* is not possible here, but the salient features of his system have seeped into many American institutions, via his students at the University of Zürich and his clinical assistants at the Burghölzli hospital.

Lombroso—Founder of Criminal Anthropology

At the close of the last century, the name of Lombroso, whether it called forth admiration or provoked an ironical smile, was to be found in many books dealing with the mental and social sciences and aroused endless discussions in student circles. For who was not familiar with the theories formulated in *L'Uomo di Genio* (*Man of Genius*), if not with those treating of differences between the white and the colored races, or in connection with woman as a delinquent?

If Lombroso is mentioned today, it is more as an eccentric. Yet his influence as a teacher and writer was great; and Italy is beholden to him for having initiated a new school in criminology, as well as for miscellaneous services to his fatherland.

Born in 1835, of poor parents, his chief absorption as a young student was linguistics, with philosophy as a side interest. Taking up Arabic, Chinese, Hebrew, and Aramaic, he might have become a comparative philologist, like his great colleague, G. I. Ascoli, but he sensed that there would be more security for him and his family if he were to study medicine. After graduation as an M.D. from the University of Padua, he began to specialize in mental disorders, a branch of medicine which had appealed to him as a student, when he wrote a long essay on the insanity of Cardano, which already contained the germ of his doctrine of degeneration.

In 1859, during the war with Austria-Hungary, he served as a medical man, and made it his hobby to study the regional types of Italy, since the soldiers came from all parts of the country. Their dialectal idiosyncrasies gave him certain clues as to their origin. What, however, catapulted the young scientist to fame was his examination of the brain of a notorious bandit who had terrorized the country before he was captured and executed. Lombroso disclosed that he shared a particular aspect of his cranium with infra-humans, namely, a furrow in the middle of the occipital lobe, found in the gorilla, chimpanzee, and other apes, but not in normal man. This led Lombroso to an extensive investigation in which he examined hundreds of skulls—those of criminals, the insane, and even, so far as they were available, of prehistoric man. His findings convinced him that there was a criminal constitution, which meant only one thing: the criminal was a throwback, an atavistic "scion" of prehistoric man.

Naturally, sociologists and social reformers, who were bending every effort to put the blame on environment, on external conditions, and on society in general, were scandalized at such an outspoken contradiction of their pet notion, and belabored him as a crackpot. He fared still worse, however, when his *Man of Genius* was published, claiming that genius is a psychical form of incipient epilepsy, and that there are definite physiological and psychic symptoms of degeneracy attending all genius.

That Lombroso's illustrations cannot be taken too seriously is recognized by anyone who reads his best-known work carefully. First, he lumps true geniuses and minor talents together. Then he adduces instances of abnormality which are hardly more than spots of sensitiveness. Pallor or some other mark of frailty represents to him a genuine stigma or constitutional defect. On top of that, he relies on anecdotes, gossip, old-wives' tales, which, in science, must be discounted. Lombroso must have caused a furor, especially in intellectual circles, where there were many who counted themselves as at least near-geniuses. At the same time, the philistines who heard of the theory —no one could expect them to read the book—must have applauded loudly, for had they not always held that there was something "crazy" about the theorist?

Actually, Lombroso was not so extreme as might be supposed. He did not contend that everyone born with criminal tendencies was bound to spend his life in crime. He made allowance for circumstances, though they were subsidiary; in other words, the criminal needed far more care than ordinary cases. But secondly, instead of appearing as the criminal's nemesis, he was able to effect certain social and legal reforms favoring the "innate" criminal, who is almost in the position of the irresponsible insane.

As to his views on genius, are they so remote from Alfred Adler's doctrine of overcompensation for a neurotic constitution or organic inferiority? Certainly, Lombroso must have credited himself with a spark of genius; hence he was not simply making goats of those we call great, while putting himself in another class. The safer conclusion is that there are geniuses and geniuses. Some are what Bleuler would call syntonic, others like Benvenuto Cellini, Villon, Van Gogh, or Blake must have had a streak of degeneracy to begin with, while others like Nietzsche and Maupassant could very well have acquired their pathological condition from toxins, infection, or the like.

Lombroso's mind was of the intuitive type, with flashes of ingenious inference illuminating a situation at intervals. He did not possess the plodding capacity of a Kraepelin. Accordingly, his patience for meticulous experimentation or critical research gave out too soon; but when he saw the connection between pellagra and the moldy corn which the peasants were eating, he became a benefactor to humanity, although his firm statement brought down the fury of the landowners upon his head.

Perhaps he will be more remembered in the annals of medical jurisprudence and criminology than as a psychiatrist. The collection of skulls and photographs which formed the nucleus of the Museum of Criminal Anthropology in Turin does credit to his industry and judgment. Among his disciples are such scholars as Enrico Ferri, Garofalo, M. Patrizi, and his son-in-law, Guglielmo Ferrero. Max Nordau's name may also be added to the list.

Some of Italy's leading psychologists have paid tribute to him as a counselor. Ferrari writes, "I went to Turin where I developed a great affection for Cesare Lombroso, a man of great genius and a great disseminator of ideas, whose criminal anthropology was beginning at last to gain favor in scientific circles," [38] while De Sanctis tells us that "many clinical and anthropological-criminal studies, which Cesare Lombroso advised me to undertake, are of this period." [39]

Max Nordau Diagnoses the Ills of Civilization

The Hungarian-born Max Simon Sudfeld (1849-1923), who is known by his *nom de plume,* Max Nordau, received his medical degree in 1875, after he had already established himself as a journalist. He was probably a good practitioner, for he had many prosperous patients, but he was more the thinker and man of letters than the medical man; and the ills which concerned him were those of society.

It is possible that his outspoken strictures were influenced by his romance with a beautiful and brilliant young American Jewess, which was shattered as a result of his mother's objection to his marrying a widow or divorcee whose modern ways, such as sending scented *billets-doux,* did not fit into the framework of a rabbinical family. The man who was to astound Europe with his straight-from-the-shoulder articulateness seemed cowed by his own mother, and the loving couple agreed to return each other's letters. The rift was apparently too much for the young woman, who opened one of her arteries in a suicide attempt. Her life was saved by the young physician from whom she had parted. The irony of the whole situation was that Nordau later married a Gentile opera singer, although certainly not to spite his mother.

Nordau's first book, which created a sensation, was called *Conventional Lies of Civilization,* published in his early thirties. To what extent Nordau went to explore the shams may be gathered from the fact that the volume was banned in Russia and in Austria. He was hardly thirty-six when his *Paradoxes* appeared, becoming a best-seller and the subject of many debates. In these books, he looms as a sociologist, with the gusto of a crusader fighting not the infidels but hypocrisy. Important as they are in their own right, their author would hardly have been more than mentioned in the present volume, but for his major work, *Degeneration.* Here he continues what Lombroso began, that is, analyzing the literary trends as well as the leading writers of the day. Dedicated to Lombroso, the book is a sort of pathography of artists, in the broad sense of the word.

The work brings out the decadent condition of the times, as Nordau saw it. His approach in dealing with the various authors is that of the alienist or clinician.

Degeneration struck like a bombshell. It was an indictment not only of Baudelaire and Verlaine, Nietzsche and Wagner, but even of men like Ruskin, Ibsen, Tolstoi, and Zola. He finds them all tainted with egomania. Ruskin may express lofty sentiments but he is "the Torquemada of aesthetics." Not only is Nordau *au courant* with the literary works of scores of authors, but he is also at home with the psychiatric contributions of Esquirol and Morel and Magnan and a host of other clinicians. Diametrically opposed as are the romanticism of a Victor Hugo and the naturalism of a Zola they have a common denominator, and Nordau cuts deep with his scalpel to lay bare the vulnerable spots in the novels, poems, plays, and short stories of the European giants. Egotism colors everything they wrote, according to him, and while he does not deny their talent in many instances, he finds them lacking in moral sensibility.

There are many passages in this extraordinarily erudite volume which might be cited, but let us confine ourselves to one which presents Nordau's psychological, and even neurological, account of degeneracy.

> Quite otherwise is the spectacle offered by the degenerate person. His nervous system is not normal. In what the digression from the norm ultimately consists we do not know. Very probably the cell of the degenerate is formed a little differently from that of sane men, the particles of the protoplasm are otherwise and less regularly disposed; the molecular movements take place, in consequence, in a less free and rapid, less rhythmic and vigorous manner. This is, however, a mere undemonstrable hypothesis. Nevertheless, it cannot reasonably be doubted that all the bodily signs or 'stigmata' of degeneration, all the arrests and inequalities of development that have been observed, have their origin in a biochemical and biomechanical derangement of the nerve-cell or, perhaps, of the cell in general.
>
> In the mental life of the degenerate, the anomaly of his nervous system has, as a consequence, the incapacity of attaining to the highest degree of development of the individual, namely, the freely coming out from the factitious limits of individuality, i.e., altruism. As to the relation of his 'Ego' to his 'non-Ego,' the degenerate man remains a child all his life. He scarcely appreciates or even perceives the external world, and is only occupied with the organic processes in his own body. He is more than egotistical, he is an egomaniac.
>
> His egomania may spring directly from dif-

ferent circumstances of his organism. His sensory nerves may be obtuse, and, in consequence, but feebly stimulated by the external world, transmit slowly and badly their stimuli to the brain, and are not in a condition to incite it to a sufficiently vigorous perceptive and ideational activity. Or his sensory nerves may work moderately well, but the brain is not sufficiently excitable, and does not perceive properly the impressions which are transmitted to it from the external world.

The obtuseness of the degenerate is attested by almost all observers.[40]

Nordau, whose sagacity and prospicience were so notable that he could predict the 1914 debacle, and whose judgment in political matters was shrewd, nevertheless did err, in the supposition that those upon whom he was passing sentence would be equally censured by posterity. Nordau, himself an intellectual of a high order, curiously enough favored the philistine as against the near-genius—an attitude which he shared with his friend Lombroso.

In Nordau's cavils there is much truth, except that they were not always directed at the proper target. They certainly applied to the decadent movement, to dadaism in art, and to the incipient expressionism of his day, but what would he have said about Gertrude Stein's verbigeration or even Joyce's lexic experiments and Dublin phantasmagorias? Above all, how would he react to the beatnik's salacious word salads which are palmed off as literature today? At the time Nordau wrote his *Degeneration,* in 1892, abstract art was not yet known. How he would have satirized the bewildering maze of lines and curves which are supposed to represent nothing visible in the picture! Nordau was neither an out-and-out radical nor a dyed-in-the-wool reactionary, but a middle-of-the-road observer. He may have been imbued with that prophetic zeal which is characteristic of spiritual leaders, but he possessed the judicial temperament, withal; and in marital devotion, paternal love, and public geniality he might be considered a paragon.

As may be surmised, Nordau's action had its reaction. In England, especially, did *Degeneration* cause bitterness. An unsigned volume under the title of *Regeneration—A Reply to Max Nordau* appeared in 1895, while G. Bernard Shaw made his rejoinder in a little book called *The Sanity of Art*. In neither was Nordau handled with kid gloves; and the anonymous one was unmistakably anti-Semitic.

In passing, it should be mentioned that without Nordau, Zionism, and thus the creation of a Jewish state, might still be only an individual longing. Theodor Herzl, who by a curious coincidence was born hardly a stone's throw from the house in Budapest where Nordau was born, sought him out in 1895 and told him that Jacob Schiff thought he was insane to toy with such a project as obtaining Palestine for the Jews. He read to the older Nordau passages from his *Altneuland*, stressing a point here and there; and after the two argued and discussed for hours on successive days, Nordau rose and with feeling embraced the younger man, saying "If you are insane, this is a case of *folie à deux;* count on me." From then on the team of Herzl and Nordau took world Jewry by storm, Herzl charming by his magnetic regal countenance and dreamy eyes, while the leonine Nordau, with his masterly rhetoric and booming voice, reminiscent of an Ezekiel of old, bidding the desiccated bones and fleshless skeletons to take on body and rise *en masse*, electrified audiences at the Zionist Congresses until they became a mass of enthusiasm, with Zion as their goal. Herzl was the man to approach rulers; Nordau negotiated the intellects and served as an intermediary for him. If Herzl was the *heart* of Zionism, Nordau was its *cortex*. Herzl gave his life for Zionism, dying at the age of forty-four, while Nordau, because of his support of Herzl on the

Uganda issue, as a temporary home for the Jews, was nearly dispatched by a bullet from a would-be assassin, a fanatical young Zionist.

Janet and the Dissociation School

Charcot's preoccupation with hysteria and the controversy between La Salpêtrière and Nancy over hypnotism and suggestion were now instrumental in moving the whole field of mental ailments away from the organic and closer to the psychological territory. It became evident, at least that perhaps procedures in attacking the subject should be reversed, and the milder disorders, which had been neglected for centuries, began to receive more attention, especially as they were more approachable and could possibly throw light on the serious manias or psychoses.

The *psychoneurosis* was beginning to grow in importance, more particularly as its extent was becoming better recognized. Although it was difficult to break away from the organic conception, acquired at such cost of energy and after such a long struggle, but stimulated by the great discoveries in the physical and natural sciences, the *psychogenic* view was beginning to gain ground. It was Pierre Janet (1859-1947), erstwhile pupil of Charcot, who took the first step, at first somewhat hesitantly, to broaden the vista. Janet, it is true, was only a sort of John the Baptist in this new movement, but thanks to his prolificacy, he was able to set up a school, until the smashing impetus of the younger Sigmund Freud took the wind out of his sails, and raised the psychological instrument to a new level.

Since Janet has already been sketched in Part I, in connection with his role as a French psychologist, we shall confine ourselves here to his contribution to abnormal psychology.

Characteristically, he was greatly interested in botany, and the herbarium which he cultivated served to remind him that human beings also constitute a kind of herbarium, containing many complex types. His uncle, the philosopher Paul Janet, was a considerable influence in his life, persuading him to take up medicine after he had already established himself as a professor of philosophy at the age of twenty-two in a lycée at Havre. It was there that he had made the acquaintance of a physician who placed at his disposal the celebrated Léonie, who, because of the experiments conducted upon her under various conditions of hypnotism, attracted the attention of a number of celebrities (Charcot, Richet) and even the British Society for Psychical Research. Léonie was said to have possessed supernormal, that is, psychic powers, but although young Janet might have suggested this as a corollary to his results, he afterward regretted the exaggerated reports and premature conclusions. Nevertheless, as early as 1882, Janet saw in Léonie a case of dissociated personality. At this time, he hadn't the slightest notion of Charcot's work, and had not even heard of Bernheim. Soon, however, he entered Charcot's laboratory, and began to publish his observations. The first mention of dissociation occurs in an article on systematized anesthesia, published in 1887.

THE PSYCHOGENIC ERA

By a stroke of coincidence, in that very same year, Freud after studying various phases of neuropathology and neurotoxology, tackled the psychological factors in mental disorders, publishing his "Beiträge zur Casuistik der Hysterie" that very same year in the *Wiener Medizinische Wochenschrift.* We may regard 1886, then, as a banner year for psychology; for it was then that the foundation was laid for the psychogenic view of disturbances that had hitherto been ascribed to organic conditions.

Janet was among the first to show the effect of suggestion on the course of hysteria (1892), and that fixed ideas aggravated the condition. He studied such states and conditions as phobias, anxiety, obsessions, various abnormal impulses, and tics. This was the day of the psychoneuroses, and Janet instituted the division of neurasthenia and psychasthenia. The first includes what we would call "jangled nerves," with symptoms such as too ready fatigability, depression, loss of appetite, clammy hands, and similar common manifestations. Loss of energy in the nerve cells is one explanation of neurasthenia, which etymologically means "nerve-weakening," so the neurological basis is not altogether to be disregarded.

In psychasthenia we have something more serious, because the deficiency is not merely that of the nerve-cells, but a loss in mental organization, dependent on deeper factors over a larger spread. Hence, the more troublesome obsessions, phobias, distortions in memory, feelings of inadequacy merging into feelings of emptiness, aboulias, conflicts, etc., which again must be separated from such conditions as epilepsy or hysteria, come under this head.

In deciding upon the etiology of the two different syndromes which characterize neurasthenia and psychasthenia, Janet points to the *degree of psychological tension* and the *particular mental level*, that is, whether on the fully conscious or the automatic, as the determinants. The weakening in the brain centers will proceed accordingly.

Janet, like Freud, did not go out of his way to account for the psychological phenomenon via physiological processes. His chief service lay in his descriptive material. He was not the systematizer that Freud was, and he did not rest content with purely psychological terms. Tending toward a physicalistic methodology, he wanted to describe even the conscious processes in objective fashion. Hence his adoption of a concept like "conduct psychology," which is close to, although not quite the same as, behaviorism. To Janet conduct psychology (which in English, at least, could be confused with the psychological propaedeutic of ethics) is superior to behaviorism, in that it permits of a hierarchy of tendencies in accordance with degrees of complexity, integration, and order of acquisition of function, so that under stress, the structure can be studied as it is beginning to give way.

Prior to the Freudian domination, Janet was looked up to as the successor of Charcot, although he lacked his dramatic personality and influence as a teacher. Janet's publications comprise more than a score of major works, several of them in two or three volumes. His chief works are *Les Névroses et les Idées fixes*, *Les Obsessions et la Psychasthénie*, *Les Médications Psychologiques*, *De l'Angoisse et l'Extase*, and *l'Evolution Psychologique de la Personnalité*. Although not a clinician or hospital director, as were his celebrated

French predecessors, he clung pretty much to the French tradition of placing therapy above all else. In the *Médications*, he intimates that so long as the patient is relieved from his distress, it matters little what method is adopted. Even quackery is to be condoned, if it works.

It is strange that Janet left no pupils in France, although he created a school which was taken quite seriously in Boston, U.S.A. As he returned to psychology in advanced age, it is almost pathetic to note that he was beginning to resort to intuition as a guide to his "conduct psychology." To an operationist or physicalist, it might seem like a case of the blind leading the lame. Janet was not blessed with the gift of a global perspective, and that was probably his bane as a scientist.

From a letter to the present author, written shortly before his death, in his eighty-sixth year, one may glean something of the vitality and drive of the founder of the Dissociation School and dean of European psychopathology during the second quarter of our century.

Morton Prince—Pioneer of Abnormal Psychology

It was in the United States that Janet had his followers; and the most prominent of them was Morton Prince (1854-1929), who had been sufficiently interested in philosophy to write a little book on psychical monism when he was scarcely out of college. As a physician, he became a disciple of Weir Mitchell ("rest cure"), but after a short stay in Paris and Nancy, he began to see the subject of nervous disorders in a new light. Impregnated with the ideas of the Dissociation School, he attached himself, in principle, to Janet and his teachings. In the United States, Prince may be considered the pioneer in abnormal psychology, to which he gave a definitely dynamic turn, early in the century. In a sense, he may be regarded as the collaborator of Freud, for whom he entertained a good deal of respect.

Prince's concept of the coconscious is not altogether remote from Freud's unconscious. His doctrine of meaning, as set forth in the first chapter of *Clinical and Experimental Studies in Personality,* is the counterpart of Freud's system of complexes, and is one of the most valuable contributions toward the understanding not only of abnormal but also of normal occurrences.

His conception of purpose, while avowedly akin to McDougall's hormic notion, is also more in line with Freud's exposition of the interplay between the individual's *superego* and the experiences which go to make up the *id,* and affect it so powerfully. Prince's reasoning does not sound so novel because he always endeavored to employ existing terms, and to bring his data into accord with accepted principle.

It is to his credit that in his search for explanations, he did not, even in those early days, move, so to speak, in a psychical vacuum. In spite of his metaphysical commitment to the idea that the ultimate essence of matter was psychic (psychical monism), he insisted on a psychophysical foundation in everything pertaining to the mind. His concept of the neurogram, as a system of neural processes (synaptic connections) where memories are stored up, which lend themselves to various degrees of activation, is not only interesting, but seems to be a sound hypothesis in accounting for most types of human behavior.

Prince was farsighted enough to sense the direction psychology would take a generation later, when he rejected the generally accepted tenet that only what is conscious, what we are aware of, is appropriate psychological subject matter (Wundt, Titchener, Münsterberg). At the same time, he was realistic enough to ground his inference in physiological, or rather neurological, concepts, often using analogies from physical theory (electron, proton) to clarify his procedure.

In all his professional vicissitudes, Prince managed to steer clear of the mechanistic whirlpool. Not that he believed in the absoluteness of introspection. The observation of objective behavior was to him a *sine qua non* of science, but the patient's testimony surely had to be taken into account. In one sense, he went beyond Janet, who influenced his line of inquiry; for he was not satisfied with halfway explanations like "incompleteness" or "exhaustion." Prince was anxious to apply the experimental method to abnormal cases. The result was that in some of his findings, he affords us significant material toward the understanding of personality.

In a number of investigations, he came upon results which show him to be an ally of Pavlov and the conditioned-reflex school. The article on "Association Neuroses," originally published in 1891, gives us the analogue of the conditioned-reflex principle applied to psychoneurotic patients. Yet the subjective factor, which is excluded by animal objectivists and behaviorists, is not eliminated from Prince's study. On the contrary, it is utilized to integrate hysterical patients whose afflictions appear not to be organic.

The artificiality of the division between the normal and the abnormal was recognized by Prince several decades ago. He dealt with conflict in a truly dynamic manner, making it virtually the property of every mental process, similar to inhibition. To be sure, he did not treat it in the grand style of Freud, who was neither hampered by psychological knowledge, nor influenced by his physiological training, but Prince's task was to supply a physical basis for the mental phenomenon.

Prince and Freud

Prince differed from Freud, in that while Freud was an affective dynamist, Prince was ideational—a relic from the ideogenic theory of his French contemporaries. If the source of the trouble is originally an unfortunate autosuggestion or induced belief, then a process of re-education is necessary to exorcise this devil. Prince's technique was based on strategy or diplomacy, at which he was a past master. He once told the author that all he would say to a wealthy hypochondriac who came to see him periodically was: "Aw, you're a damn fool! That's all." The patient would laugh uproariously and then hand him fifty dollars. But Prince could have said the few words so charmingly and jovially that the abuse served as therapy.

Prince's adventures into the awesome realm of multiple personality produced something of a stir. His *Dissociation of a Personality* read like fiction; and some of his colleagues regarded it as close to it. But the lady in question, who was by no means a questionable lady (she later married a prominent colleague of Prince) did go through a number of split stages. Without at the time knowing the relationship —I happened to ask her husband why there were practically no cases of double or multiple personality in our own generation, and was told that actually there are, but that they are not drawn out because professional interest has shifted to other problems and phenomena.

Because of his social standing, contacts, and means, Prince was able to consolidate the workers in psychopathology. He founded the *Journal of Abnormal Psychology*, arranged symposia (*e.g.*, on the subconscious), was largely instrumental in getting Janet as chief speaker at the dedication of the new Harvard Medical School, and in having McDougall invited to fill the chair of William James in the Harvard psychology department. After leaving Tufts University, he gave courses at Harvard and founded the Harvard Psychological Clinic.

Among moments to be remembered are the meetings of the "Olympians" in Prince's house on 376 Beacon Street, Boston, where entomologist Wheeler, biologist Henderson, physiologist Cannon, psychiatrist Myerson, and a few psychologists (of which the present writer was the youngest) would discuss after a Welsh rabbit, in an atmosphere of gracious living, the problems common to all. To commemorate his seventieth anniversary the author brought out a *Festschrift* (*Problems of Personality*), each of its contributors being, with one or two exceptions, distinguished men—Janet, McDougall, Jung, Ernest Jones, Jelliffe, G. Elliot Smith, W. A. White, Mills, Charles L. Dana, Ramsey Hunt, Macfie Campbell, Charles S. Myers (Cambridge), William Brown (Oxford), Goddard, and MacCurdy. No mention of his age was made in the volume. The present author brought together Prince's more important papers in clinical psychology and personality under the title of *Clinical and Experimental Studies in Personality* (second enlarged edition, 1939, Sci-Art). His book *The Unconscious,* in which he develops his theory of the coconscious, is practically a textbook in psychology, along structural (Wundt, Titchener) lines.

Prince took an active part in international politics and was decorated by the Japanese Emperor. A special Prince room, containing his library and many relics, has been set apart in the Boston Medical Library.

Adolf Meyer and Psychobiology

In 1892, there came to the United States a young Swiss immigrant by the name of Adolf Meyer (1866-1950), who had studied at Zürich, Paris, London, Edinburgh, and Berlin. Before settling at Johns Hopkins University, he was director of research at various hospitals and taught psychiatry at Cornell University (1904-1909). At Johns Hopkins, in Baltimore, he served as professor of psychiatry from 1910 to 1941, and part of this period as Director of the Phipps Psychiatric Clinic.

Unlike Kraepelin or Janet, he did not turn out a mass of literature. His output, in fact, was remarkably small. An edition of fifty-two papers, brought out by one of his students (Lief), constituted the bulk of his work. Not even a simple textbook came from his pen, and yet he was held in high regard by his colleagues both here and abroad, receiving many honors.

Several reasons may be assigned for this. In the first place, he was a stimulating teacher and a man whose personal dignity counted for more than an ambition to stir the world. Of a serious mien, he never took himself too seriously, but upon a first meeting would try to understand his interlocutor rather than study him, thus giving the impression of a becoming modesty. Furthermore, although he was opposed to the systems of Kraepelin, Freud, and Janet (if the latter can be said to have had a system), he never engaged in polemics.

Meyer is not noted for any special theories or new coinages which might serve as rallying points for a closely knit school. He did use the term "mental hygiene" for the first time, and with the aid of Clifford Beers (*The Mind That Found Itself*) he sparked the movement that soon outgrew its original purpose. He also initiated the trend which he denominated "Psychobiology," to the extent of inducing, perhaps indirectly, Knight Dunlap, the head of the psychology department at Johns Hopkins, to publish a slender textbook on the subject. No doubt he was also sympathetic to John Watson's objective outlook, although he did not approve of his extreme behaviorism. Differing from most psychiatrists, he was abreast of what was going on in psychology, contributing not infrequently to psychological periodicals. Among his noted students were F. Ebaugh, C. Macfie Campbell, and W. Muncie, who succeeded him at Johns Hopkins.

Common Sense Approach in Psychiatry

Meyer was closer in temperament and conception to the French clinicians prior to Charcot, than to the Germans. The *whole individual* was important to him and not merely the symptoms or the disease. He was less anxious to discover general laws than to treat each patient in accordance with his own circumstances. Past experiences are, of course, significant, but so are the events of the present. As a functionalist, he concerned himself with the adaptational capacities in relation to the aspirations of the patient. The activities of the individual as a whole come under the head of what he called "ergasiology." Thus, he approaches Adler's views, on the one hand, and Goldstein's organismic picture, on the other.

Constitutional factors, like instinctual drives, individual rhythms, allergies, capacities, efficiency level, and intelligence potential, are balanced against acquired skills, habits, moods, visions, aspirations, memories of the past, and present associations. As Muncie puts it, "Medical men, dealing with both personality functions and the workings of organ systems have a unique opportunity of observing human behavior, living out the events of a biography with their personal and social implications. When this biography is attended with a degree of orderly operation and satisfaction from life, it is called normal."[41]

Meyer's procedure, then, was to interpret in terms of overt behavior and not through a postulated set of unconscious mechanisms or a hypothetical lesion of some tissue. He was no speculator, but a conservative investor; for to him starting with a theory of a universal nature would mean that the therapist could, in his bias and enthusiasm, be led astray and overlook the actual source of the trouble. He, therefore, proposed to approach the patient with an open mind, prepared to receive cues from the unfolding of the case after all the required data had been gathered under strict control.

Certainly there was nothing flamboyant about such a system, yet Meyer came to be looked upon as the Dean of American psychiatry, and was much sought after in the council halls of psychiatric administrators, who respected his seasoned judgment. It was evident that here was a man who knew more than his writings indicated. At our first meeting, in Cambridge, toward the end of his life, he surprised the writer by telling him that it was he who had ordered most of his books for the Johns Hopkins Library. At the most, it might have been expected that only the name of this psychologist would be familiar to him, but Meyer avowed reading many of his works.

In a private communication, the animal psychologist, R. M. Yerkes, related an episode which revealed a characteristic Meyer trait. To celebrate Meyer's anniversary, a number of his colleagues and former students, aware of his aversion to being fêted and also knowing of his temperance sympathies, thought up the ruse of inviting him to a prohibition meeting, which, in reality, turned out to be a dinner in his honor—minus the drinks, of course. My correspondent did not divulge just how Meyer took the little conspiracy.

Freud—The Era of Depth Psychology
The Man Who Revolutionized the Mental Sciences

The thinking of three men dominates the modern world, each one having taken for his domain a special sector of knowledge.

Karl Marx, the economic and political theorist, divided the world into two large ideologies espoused by two opposing global camps; and although he operated in the economic sphere, his conclusions pointed to an all-embracing philosophy of historical determinism which colored the whole social fabric. As this was embraced by zealots who were concerned with propaganda and conquest rather than with theoretical issues and specific applications, its implications were factitiously extended to all human endeavor, including even the natural and physical sciences.

Albert Einstein's sovereignty in the domain of science is of a narrower compass, but its hold is far more established. His formulas are now unquestioned.

Another thinker of the same period, Sigmund Freud, set his stamp on modern civilization, to an even greater extent than either of the other two, and whether or not one accepts his system as a whole, even his opponents must recognize that he has broadened our intellectual horizon, and that both psychology and psychopathology have taken a new turn largely through his exploratory genius. Freud definitely broke with the past, paradoxically enough, by emphasizing the past of every individual, thus transcending the merely psychogenic station of Janet's Dissociation School, and setting up a tridimensional structure for the understanding of man, which he called "psychoanalysis."

Psychoanalysis has permeated every cultural endeavor within the last few decades: medicine, art, fiction, drama, biography, literary criticism, and even history. Without Freud, Eugene O'Neill's dramas would not have been the same. As to history, a former President of the American Historical Association (Langer) has declared: "Psychoanalysis has long ceased being merely a therapy and has been generally recognized as a theory basic to the study of the human personality. . . . Clearly the time has come for us to reckon with a doctrine that strikes so close to the heart of our own discipline."

Freud did not, as is sometimes supposed, discover the unconscious. Leibniz, Schopenhauer, Hartmann and F. C. Myers (who, by the way, was the one to liken the unconscious to the submerged part of an iceberg, an analogy attributed to Freud) were his predecessors. Still less may it be said that he discovered sex. He merely illuminated it, just as he made us very conscious of the unconscious, and relegated the conscious, which had been the exclusive subject matter of psychology, to a secondary place.

He took cognition down from its laboratory pedestal in academic psychology, and in its place he enthroned affection or feeling. Another break with scientific psychology was his preoccupation with the "why" or "wherefore," whereas all his predecessors had been busily engaged searching for the "how" in physiological terms, so as to establish laws. Trained in neurology, he nevertheless was not overawed by its discipline and dared to erect a psychological edifice quite independent of any physiological foundation—at least for the present. To him, not the *cause* but the *motive* was important in the human sphere; and brain cells or nerve fibers can tell us nothing about motives.

Thus Freud stepped from one ledge to another outside the traditional framework, pointing up the role of the irrational as against the rational and logical in our behavior, from which it follows that there is only an imaginary boundary between the normal and the abnormal. If the unconscious determines our acts, it is only reasonable to suppose that they are not governed by reason; for the unconscious is *eo ipso* outside of our rational control.

The significance of trifles is another of Freud's findings which went against the grain in conventional circles; and as if these heresies were insufficient, he even went so far as to espouse the view that psychic energy can be transformed into physical, *e.g.*, in the case of hysterical pain which ceases and turns into depression, or vice versa. Such an hypothesis is unacceptable in science.

However, what made Freud's name a byword of disreputableness was not so much his reversal of received beliefs, his upsetting of the psychological applecart, as his making out of the innocent babe a sensual lover of the parent of the opposite sex. Indeed that fixation—the Oedipus complex in the boy and the Electra complex in the girl at a very tender age—is in reality the prop of the whole system, and the root of all the quirks and kinks of the later neurotic, who by virtue of his stumped genitality is still lingering at the oral or the anal, or urethral, or phallic level of libido development. Thus the bothersome complexes in the unconscious, which are reactivated by recent occurrences, break through in hysteria, perversions, and various kinds of psychoneuroses like phobias, anxieties, and depressions.

His division of the mind topographically into (a) the *id* (the reservoir of pleasure impulses); (b) the ego (the system of realistic tendencies making for stability and social status); and (c) the superego (the matrix of conscience and scrupulousness) all ties up with the doctrine of genital development.

A strict determinism or even an overdeterminism, as when several submotives are at work, renders interpretation simple so that everyone trained in psychoanalysis will eventually come to the same conclusion. Therapy consists in bringing the complexes to the fore and breaking the patient's resistance to discerning the culprits underneath.

Freud the Man

Sigmund Freud was born in Freiberg, Moravia, in 1856, of Jewish parents who migrated to Vienna, where he was educated. After graduation from the University of Vienna, he went to Paris, as a physician, where he attended the lectures of Charcot, in 1885, and also visited Nancy, coming under the influence of Bernheim, whose book on suggestion he translated into German, adding a lengthy introduction of his own.

As Josef Breuer's assistant, young Freud was struck with the stalling of a patient (who happened to be the later famous Bertha Pappenheim) in presenting the crucial facts of her case. Hypnosis seemed to be of some service; and after repeated and insistent questioning by Breuer, she was able to relate a mass of facts; and the unburdening herself of certain incidents relating to her hysterical condition stemming from a sense of guilt in connection with her father's death (fairly common among devoted children) was thought to have effected her cure. Thus was Anna O., as Freud named her in the literature, instrumental in ushering in the psychoanalytic era. She was, however, more important in her own right; for she subsequently became one of the worthiest women in Germany, the Bonn Government issuing a commemorative stamp in her honor. The present writer's *Freudiana* is dedicated to her memory.

But psychoanalysis is pertinent not only in the treatment of ailments. It purports to explain the origin of wit and myths, to interpret dreams, to account for artistic impulses, and even religious tendencies. In fact, it undertakes to examine the whole fabric of civilization with its fluoroscope and to reduce all social and cultural phenomena to one common denominator—the love urge, in its countless transformations and disguises. To this purpose, the journal *Imago* was founded, and later one of its editors, Hanns Sachs, on settling in Boston, founded *The American Imago,* which still publishes interesting speculations on cultural matters.

Freud's books have sold in the millions in numerous languages. His most widely read are *Introduction to Psychoanalysis* (2nd Series), *Interpretation of Dreams, Wit and the Unconscious, Psycho-*

pathology of Everyday Life, Leonardo da Vinci, Totem and Tabu, Civilization and Its Discontents and *Moses and Monotheism.*

His life, from the time he published his *Interpretation of Dreams,* in fact, even after the appearance of his and Breuer's book on the role of sex in hysteria, was one vast struggle. At first he fought poverty, then he wrestled with the problems of his own circle of followers, some of whom became dissidents, while others were, like children, divided by jealousy, envy, soaring ambitions, personality clashes. His aggravated mouth cancer and the multiple operations necessitating the use of mechanical gadgets made his lot even more trying. But the abuse heaped upon him by the official defenders of tradition was, as his doctrines began to spread, gradually counterbalanced by the favor that came to him after his invitation by Stanley Hall to be chief guest at the Clark University Commemorative exercises, in 1909.

The most gripping act of the Freud drama came when the Nazi monster, on annexing Austria, turned to its prize prey, who might have ended up, like his sisters, in gas chamber and crematory, were it not for the feverish efforts of devoted friends in high office, and principally the decisive maneuver of his disciples, Ernest Jones and Princess Marie Bonaparte, who spirited him out of Vienna to Paris, from where he went to London, where he died just before the Nazi war broke out.

Freud was fortunate in his biographer, Ernest Jones, who devoted ten years and three large volumes of some seventeen hundred pages to tell the story. The Freud cinema, especially since at least half of Hollywood's stardom has been psychoanalyzed, promises to be one of the most absorbing productions ever seen on the screen, exemplifying the dictum that "truth is stranger than fiction." Indeed, the more documentary the film, in this case, the greater its value as a work of art, since the Nazis have already provided the explosive ingredients. Thus Freud not only is a lonely explorer, a controversial scientist, a psychologist-rebel, a healer, but also looms as a historical symbol, a forced actor in the spectacle of the twentieth-century Middle Ages.

Jung and Analytic Psychology

Freud's most brilliant associate was Carl Gustav Jung (1875-1961), with roots in Basel and Zürich, the scion of a cultured ancestry, including parsons, a surgeon, and other academic men. Jung's early interests were in the biological sciences, but apparently one part of him was constantly drawn to philosophy, religion, mythology, and the occult. If he decided to take up medicine, it was more for practical reasons, for he always remained the humanist burrowing along side paths and, like Freud, exploring among the débris of abandoned views and little-known doctrines.

Jung had become partial to Freud's novel system as early as the turn of the century, when he was writing his doctoral dissertation on the psychology and pathology of so-called occult phenomena, a subject which he has dwelt on persistently in his latest productions. The word-association experiments which brought Jung his early prestige were also linked up with psychoanalysis. Jung became attached to Freud, while Freud showed an almost paternal affection for the handsome, urbane, imaginative young physician. In less than seven years, 330 letters were exchanged between them, although the latter ones were scarcely in character with their early relationship.

Jung became a close collaborator of Freud, one of the editors of the psychoanalytic periodicals, and, it would seem, was highly favored by the chief. In 1909 he accompanied Freud to America. In 1912, to the chagrin of Freud's critical lieutenants, Jung became President of the International Psychoanalytic Association. But alas, never was the couplet so true that "East is East and West is West," for although the twain did meet, they met only to part company. Jung could not stomach the incest theory of Freud. He used the word "libido" too; but he did not attach to it a sexual connotation. His "libido" was similar to Bergson's *"élan"* or the horme which McDougall adopted. To this day, he shows his indebtedness to the Founder, although there have been times when his aggressiveness and resentment moved him to make certain statements about Freud's almost exclusively Jewish patients and associates which could be interpreted as anti-Semitic. In reality, Jung, whose chief goal has been to discover the contents of the collective unconscious, which he postulated, is convinced that there are different archetypes for different ethnic stocks, and that the Germans and the Jews do not share a common mode of thought because their archetypes—i.e., patterns of the collective unconscious symbolizing a particular group or era—are disparate.

These archetypes are manifested in dreams, among other phenomena, and Jung contends that Freud's particularly sexual inferences are possible only in the light of Jewish dreams. Among the most important archetypes are such image concepts as "the devil" or the "animus," i.e., the mate-ideal in the female psyche, and conversely the "anima" or mate-ideal in the male psyche. Myths and children's imaginings are all considered emanations of the collective unconscious.

Jung is committed to the doctrine that the unconscious of the individual, which begins with infant experiences, is grafted onto a much vaster unconscious, the experiences of the race, hence for him Freud's psychoanalysis does not go back far enough. Freud, the rationalist, although deriving from some of his mystic forebears, was schooled in the tenets of an enlightenment philosophy. At times, he, too, evinces the influence of the occult, and on occasion, he betrays a hankering for a collective memory ingrained in the racial psyche, but he prefers to avoid speculating without the prospect of inducing conviction through reasonable evidence. Jung, it would seem, is prepared to appeal to our very sense of the collective unconscious, to our very archetype itself.

In addition, while Freud was bred (not necessarily at home) in an atmosphere of agnosticism, Jung is essentially of a religious nature. Freud's ethical relativity is foreign to Jung. The latter sees in neurosis a lack of wholesomeness, and therefore a need for moral elevation. In that respect, Jung is not too far removed from Heinroth (*q.v.*) or Dubois his Swiss predecessor. Let it not be assumed that Jung has been more ethical than Freud. We are here simply on theoretical ground. One can well understand why a man like William McDougall, equally inclined toward religion, the occult and taking stock in the generally discarded view of the transmission of acquired characteristics, would go to Jung for his psychoanalytic training rather than to Freud, who, in his eyes, tended to degrade the human soul.

Jung could not, even had he wished to, apply the term "psychoanalysis" to his system, and so he designated it "analytic psychology." He might well have called it "psychosynthesis," for in straightening out his patient, he claims to be putting him together by making him understand the situation not in terms of mechanisms and complexes but in the full perspective.

Of the score or more of books which Jung has published, probably his most suggestive is *Wandlungen und Symbole der Libido* (*Transformations and Symbols of the Libido*), 1912. His most important is that on *Psychological Types*. His division of humans into introverts and extraverts is popularly known and requires no exposition here. What is not generally known, perhaps not even by Jung himself, is that the terms "introversion" and "extraversion" were used by others, prior to him, in practically the same context.

Jung, possibly because of his address and bearing, has been successful in contacts with the wealthy. He has visited the United States several times. At the Harvard Tercentenary, he was awarded an honorary doctorate together with Janet. After the Hitler war, his visit to America was prevented by an outcry to the effect that he had been close to the Nazis. Some even went so far as to maintain that he had been called out to treat Hitler. It may be true that he nurtured some slight admiration for Hitler as an almost infallibly intuitive mind, but he denied in a letter to the present author that he sympathized with the Nazi ideology. Indeed, he felt that Hitler was a danger—but then states are monsters, anyway.

Jung's erudition is extraordinary. Even Ernest Jones, who was his antipode both officially and temperamentally, pays tribute to his lively imagination. In his eighty-sixth year he is still intellectually active, bringing out new books or revising the old ones. Almost every intelligent reader can profit from them, but it takes the romantic to accept the majority of his hypotheses and formulations. In England, H. G. Baynes devoted most of his later years to spreading Jung's gospel, both through translations and expositions.

Adler and Individual Psychology

Another rebel who was strongly influenced at the meetings of the Vienna Psychoanalytic Society was Alfred Adler (1870-1937). Born in a suburb of Vienna, he received his medical degree from the University in 1895. In 1902, he joined Freud's circle, and because of his periodical contributions, which were drawing attention in professional quarters, he was looked up to as a leader until the advent of Jung.

Adler, however, was already beginning to swerve to the right. It was reported that he once protested against having to stand in the shadow of Freud. The final break came in 1911, when as President of the Vienna Society, he began to outline his own principles which were in contravention of those laid down by Freud. In the first place, belief in the sexual source of all human drives, as presented in orthodox psychoanalysis, did not appear valid to him. Nor did he believe that the unconscious was the all-in-all. Not only would he flout such a concept as a "collective unconscious," which was pivotal to Jung, but most of the Freudian mechanisms had little significance for him. Nevertheless, Freud might have made allowance for such heresies, had not some of his more dogmatic disciples pointed out that the name of the Society would have to be changed in order to incorporate Adler's ideas into its program and framework. Adler was then ousted, and promptly started a school of his own which he called *Individual Psychology*—not a felicitious designation since it gives rise to the misunderstanding that the dichotomy was between *individual* and *collective* psychology, whereas actually the term has reference to the fact that Adler proposed to treat the *whole individual,* and not a bundle of complexes.

Organ Inferiority and Compensation

What did Adler substitute for the all-powerful libido of psychoanalysis? Taking his cue from Nietzsche and the French moralists, he decided that the driving motive in human life was the goal of superiority; as a psychiatrist he could observe the many occasions on which this goal is thwarted, and he came to the conclusion that such frustrations provided the makings of a neurotic. Since, however, every person is bound to find obstacles in his way, it is incumbent upon us to account for the causes which operate in the succumbing to or surmounting of them.

Abreast of the psychiatric literature of the day, Adler suggested that the psychic weakness lay in organic inferiority or in its governing factor in the upper nervous system. Women are burdened with added constitutional disabilities, so that there develops in many of them a masculine protest which provokes a hostile attitude in others, which, in its turn, produces bitterness, and thus the vicious circle leads to deeper neurosis.

Since, however, there are some comparatively nonneurotic people, and also many who have made their neurosis work for society, the problem is not solved until we find another agency which accounts for the differences. Adler did not have to go far to discover it. It was something which had been known through the ages—the mechanism of *compensation*. In physiology, vicarious functioning in the case of the impairment of one part of a double organ was an elementary fact, but G. Anton, in 1906, writing on the compensation of function in cerebral disease, brought in the concept of "psychical transplantation." The cowardice of neurotics, e.g., he believes to be a species of defense mechanism. Hysteria, similarly, can be a protection against the ravaging consequence of grief, or mortification; and an attitude of apathy is assumed by a neurotic who is prone to flare up, to his undoing.[42]

Freud himself made much of the compensation principle, and Adler extended the doctrine in a new direction: The nonneurotic, if there is such, has compensated adequately for his constitutional inferiority; the neurotic has failed to make such adjustment; while the genius has overcompensated in a manner which proves serviceable to the world.

Adler's book on the neurotic constitution and his larger work, *The Practice and Theory of Individual Psychology,* were scientific treatises which incorporated many clinical observations. It was not long, however, before he took a sociological approach and shifted his emphasis to what he dubbed the "style of life." The neurosis or tension is now seen as the result of the relationship of parent to child, and of child to sibling. It makes all the difference in the world whether the individual is an only child, the first, the second, third, or last in a specific family.

When he arrived in the United States in 1926, he began to open child clinics (since in Vienna he had been entrusted with directing the first clinic for juvenile delinquents) and toured the country making much headway. Adler was visiting professor at Columbia University in 1928-1929, and from 1932 to 1937 he taught at the Long Island Medical School.

Adler's subsequent books, such as *Understanding Human Nature* (1927), *The Science of Living* (1929), and *Educating Children* (1930), are popular not only in style but in range of conception. It seems to many that his earlier work was more original and more solid.

Nevertheless Adler had many followers. Phyllis Bottome has written a full-length biography of him, while a periodical devoted to "individual psychology" is still enjoying some circulation. Adler's name is generally associated with the term "inferiority complex," but he favored rather such states as "feeling," i.e., the conscious rather than unconscious mechanisms, like complexes.

Adler's star has been in the ascendant with para-Freudians, who have come to see Freud's deficiency in placing mechanisms and complexes above character and self-discipline. It is evident that Adler stressed the reality principle, as against the *id* and the *superego* in Freud's topographical economy. Freud was beginning to shift emphasis too, but he did not live long enough to carry through. Adler was more self-deterministic than Freud, so that many educators were disposed to accept his teachings in preference to Freud's. Adler made much of understanding the patient, which strikes a sympathetic chord in many professionals today. While Freud rejected the organic or somatic conceptions of mental disease, he still clung to the impersonal technique of probing mechanisms.

It was not because of Adler that many analysts have strayed of late from the orthodox fold and begun to dwell on the ego principle which is the nubbin of Adler's psychology. It is merely the return swing of the pendulum after it has gone beyond the legitimate point in the arc.

WILHELM STEKEL (1860-1940)

If Stekel's brand of psychoanalysis is not discussed here more fully, it is not because of neglect but rather for the reason that Stekel was an eclectic and, although perhaps the most brilliant interpreter of all of Freud's disciples, he never established himself on a wholly independent footing, as did Jung and Adler. If the others might be conceived as composers, he was more the great virtuoso in execution. It may be said of him, however, that his polyphonic interpretations of dreams, in which he excelled, did make allowance for a characterial phase, which he called the *functional* as opposed to the *material* content that involved the pure *id;* and thus Silberer's distinction of anagogic (elevating) and catagogic ("gutterward") found its way into his psychological outlook, drawing Freud's barbed shafts in consequence.

Many of Stekel's works have been translated into English. These include *Compulsion and Doubt* (2 vols.), *Frigidity in Women* (2 vols.), *Peculiarities of Behavior* (2 vols.), *Interpretation of Dreams* (2 vols.), *Sadism and Masochism, The Beloved Ego* and *Disguises of Love.*

In observing symbolism in human behavior, Stekel has the edge on Freud. He sees masked sex or its sublimation in almost every action. If a woman cannot make up her mind in buying hats, it is because she has made a poor choice in her husband. The well-known dread of getting in the dentist's chair (years ago, when teeth were pulled not so painlessly) to Stekel bespeaks an unconscious fear on the part of the fiancé that his love has no real *roots*. A collector of stamps, buttons, flowers or what-not is a derailed Don Juan, while if you are late for an appointment, you are betraying submerged resentment for being born after other children in the family and thus missing the opportunities enjoyed by those born earlier.

His dream books teem with sexual references, especially in relation to the mechanism of the automobile. He is, withal, a fascinating entertainer and a sophisticate who writes well, if not convincingly. Whether he is more suggestive than stimulating is a moot point, but he stresses, certainly more than Freud, the anagogic—that is, the "upward-leading" —in dreams, and injects moral values into the treatment.

OTTO RANK (1884-1939)—Freud's Favorite Rebel

Otto Rank was ousted from the orthodox group in Vienna when he elevated the birth trauma, which Freud originally suggested in a casual way, into a psychoanalytic fetish. That such an unknowable factor could be the basis of all neurosis is almost incomprehensible. But there were other signs of rebelliousness in the youngest of Freud's heirs, for he advocated a condensed form of analysis, which would take only weeks, or at most months, instead of years. Rank was a prodigious worker, endowed with the fervor, undisciplined cultural sweep, and power of synthesis usually found in the East European, Talmudical scholar. In his large work on the incest motive in literature, he did yeoman's service for his master. All his books, however, are marked by flashes of originality. Inevitably, he reminds us of another Otto—Otto Weininger, who committed suicide at the age of twenty-three, after achieving a phenomenal success with his *Sex and Character*. In his *Myth of the Birth of the Hero* (Nervous and Mental Disease Monographs, No. 18) Rank expresses the opinion that schizophrenia results from a conflict between the masculine and feminine elements in a personality. This is what Weininger might have concluded, had he reached a mature age.

Rank's therapy consisted mainly in causing the patient to re-experience the birth trauma, something which Freud, for valid reasons, could not countenance. In the United States, where Rank spent his last few years, he found The Pennsylvania School of Social Work, about the only place where his methods were adopted, and where the patient found his task almost one of penance. No wonder his last work was called *Will Therapy,* and that is the name his method goes by among social workers.

Rank's emphasis on will therapy takes him further away from his master and brings him closer to Dubois, the Swiss practitioner. Indeed, he even outdoes him in severity of discipline.

In his comparatively short life, wracked with pain and borne down with mental anguish toward the end, Rank published more than a dozen works, some of them of great scope. His *Incest Motif in Fiction and Legend* was greatly admired by Freud. It has never appeared in English. Among his other books are *The Don Juan Figure, Psychology and the Soul Technique of Psychoanalysis; Myth of the Birth of the Hero; History of the Human Will; Art and Artist; Will Therapy; Truth and Reality in Life; Foundations of a Genetic Psychology.*

CLINICAL MORPHOLOGY—KRETSCHMER

The psychoanalytic movement has done much to undermine the somatic and organic conceptions of mental disease, for if the early childhood experiences in connection with the libido (including excretory functions) form character and are instrumental in the later development of neuroses and/or the channeling of creative impulses, then the congenital constitution of the individual must be of little consequence, especially as, in accordance with Freudian premises, the sex experiences of all children follow pretty much the same pattern.

It is fortunate, however, for the growth of science that no trend enjoys a complete monopoly. There are always outstanding workers who hew to the traditional course and, even when they are not particularly concerned in demolishing what may appear to them as freak deviations, will not only succeed in preserving the *status quo* but will re-enforce it by means of freshly acquired data.

One of the latest outgrowths of the *rapprochement* between anatomy, anthropology and psychiatry is the experimental move to correlate temperament with bodily proportions. In a sense, it is an extension of physiognomy, which was never held in good repute, but since anthropology had much to do with bodily measurements, it must have helped the course of clinical morphology. De Giovanni in Italy, about 1890, began a series of investigations, continued by other Italians, which yielded a number of interesting results, such as the correlation of tall persons with the phthisic habitus (susceptibility to pulmonary ailments) and of stocky ones with the apoplectic habitus.

In France, the gastroenterist, C. Sigaud, somewhat later published his work on human morphology, which sets up four types of man, viz., the cerebral (which corresponds to the mental), the respiratory, the digestive, and the muscular, each of which is not only differently constituted *ab ovo,* but reacts differently to a similar environment. A number of his pupils, in particular L. MacAuliffe, have extended the experiments under a biochemical purview. Some have injected endocrinological considerations into their researches. It is clear that the aim of these men was to establish a schema of types which would be more reliable and serviceable than the old temperament series.

It was about the time when psychoanalysis had turned the heads of professionals in Europe and America that Ernst Kretschmer (1888-) brought out his book on *Physique and Character* (*Körperbau und Charakter*), in which Sigaud's four types are almost duplicated, but on a more solid footing. Kretschmer's four types were (a) the asthenic, (b) the pyknic, (c) the athletic, and (d) the dysplastic. Afterward the leptosome or long-bodied was substituted for the asthentic, which was made a subtype. We now see that the leptosome would correspond to Sigaud's respiratory (tubular lungs), and the pyknic (corpulent, stocky) is simply another word for the digestive, while athletic and muscular are practically synonymous. The only new type is the dysplastic, i.e., the disproportioned. Sigaud's cerebral is either leptosome or asthenic.

It was Kretschmer's belief that there were in reality two biotypes, the schizothymic and the cyclothymic, corresponding to the leptosome and the pyknic in physique. These types find their counterparts in other schemata, like Jung's introverts and extraverts,

Gross's secondary-function and primary-function classes, but the prime importance of the division is to diagnose or even predict the type of mental trouble which may develop in specific individuals of a given build. Thus the leptosome or asthenic when succumbing to stress is expected to develop symptoms of schizophrenia (dementia praecox, megalomania, paranoia, etc.), while the pyknic or stocky individual will, under similar circumstances, show signs of manic-depressive disorder.

As may be imagined, such theories found both advocates and opponents. Hundreds of papers were written in order either to prove or to disprove Kretschmer's findings. American psychologists, by and large, are loath to accept any type theory, contending that it is rare to come upon an individual who falls plump into any one of the formulated categories. What they do not perceive, apparently, is that the types include tendencies, and that it is rare for a person not to come under a *tendency* to approximate this or that type.

In the United States, an able ally to Kretschmer's theories was found in W. H. Sheldon, whose division of human beings into the ectomorph (long-bodied), mesomorph (muscular), and endomorph (corpulent), based on many thousands of measurements correlated with behavioral and clinical observations, tended to confirm Kretschmer. Each of these constitutions represents, according to Sheldon, a different combination of the cerebral, visceral, and muscular components, and if each should be arranged on a scale of seven values, then a constitution of 612 would signify a comfort-loving, corpulent person with extraverted or sociable tendencies, not interested in the intellectual life, and even less in athletics; while a 126 would reveal the tall or slim, nervous and wiry brain worker. If the tension under stress becomes unendurable, the former is potentially a manic-depressive; the latter a candidate for schizophrenia.

With the aid of assistants, Sheldon has worked out an atlas of combinations with character delineations for each one. Allowing for a good deal of unwarranted generalization, there is a wealth of material here to be utilized in practical applications, not only in psychopathology, but in correctional matters, and in personnel administration. To what extent the individual is typical of his or her sex has been made the object of further study. A strong or weak masculine component bespeaks a different setup of certain traits.

Kretschmer has had to defend himself against both psychological and medical researchers ever since his *Körperbau und Charakter* first appeared. He has had to give account of his methodology to the factorial analysts, to biologists, to anthropologists and to sundry critics who simply reject the whole idea of "type" as something antiquated. In the preface of the twenty-first edition of his best-known work, he rightly complains of the contrast assumed between morphology and functional studies; for physique is nothing more than the slow development of a series of discharging functions into a unit. By 1950, as many as 65,000 cases had been examined by Kretschmer and his associates from a number of different angles. Thus his theory is based on a formidable array of evidence.

Kretschmer's dynamic tendency had already manifested itself in his early monograph on the delusion of reference (*Der sensitive Beziehungswahn*), which appeared in 1918. The *temporal development* of the experience from its entry until its exit is to Kretschmer the crux of the situation. The *impressionability* of the individual is the first factor; then comes the retentivity, which instead of being an asset is here a liability; the intrapsychic exploitation of the experience is the most critical stage; and ultimately, the dischargeability or abreactivity will tell the final story. If that is prevented, through the asthenic character of the individual, anxiety and scrupulosity interpose, and when the condition reaches a climax, *inversion* takes place: the primary experience is inwardly directed and assimilated into a group of ideas which had been elaborated into a secondary thought mechanism, receiving undue attention and forming a little system of its own—a sort of parallel ghost train, which is only superficially associated with the real happenings.

Ernst Kretschmer was professor at Marburg but is currently at the University of Tübingen, directing the psychiatric clinics. His most important works, in addition to those already discussed, are his book on *Hysteria* (1927), *Psychology of Men of Genius* (1931), *Medical Psychology* (1939). and *Hysteria, Reflex and Instinct* (1960).

THE THERAPISTS

It may be assumed that therapy was the objective of all mental institutions and their administrators, as well as physicians, from the earliest times, but the routine treatment of patients through bleeding, purging, or diet was a slow process of rather doubtful results.

It is only in our own century that more daring methods have been resorted to; and although in theory they were suggested or presaged centuries ago, they were never carried out—for one reason, because a high level of general medical information and technique had to be reached before experimentation could be hazarded in a sphere where it was "do or die." Since the psychotic was not in the same threatening circumstances as someone suffering from a strangulated hernia or in an aggravated condition of septicemia, the urgency to take a bold step was not equally present.

Chemotherapy, especially sedation, was of course always in vogue, but nothing definite had been established so far as cure was concerned.

WAGNER-JAUREGG
and Fever Inducing

In his autobiography, the Viennese psychiatrist Julius Wagner-Jauregg (1857-1940) tells how he came upon the idea of inoculating general paretics with the blood of a soldier ill with malaria. He cites Parmenides, who exclaimed in 500 B.C., "Give me the power to produce fever and I'll cure all disease," while Hippocrates spoke of the beneficial effect of fever on epilepsy. It was, however, an observation of Francis Bacon which made a special impression on him. Bacon had written that it was essential for physicians to study the cured cases of incurable diseases, and although this seems to us an Irish bull, Wagner-Jauregg knew what it meant.

He had already shown excellent promise a few years earlier in his experimental studies on the thyroid gland and cretinism; and now as a young assistant, in 1883, he began to investigate those cases of mental illness which had been practically cured after accidental infection. He noticed that a psychotic woman became practically normal after a siege of erysipelas.

Wagner-Jauregg made many experiments with injections of various kinds, even tuberculin, and in most cases obtained satisfactory results, but he could not establish whether the cure might not have come even without the inoculation. It was a few cases of general paresis which decided the matter; for this disease was regarded definitely as incurable. Wagner-Jauregg, after trying out various vaccines, decided on one inducing typhus, and with added mercury and iodine and thence neosalvarsan, which Ehrlich had just made available, proceeded to make medical history. But his reports at medical congresses received an indifferent reception, and even as late as 1912, comments in standard textbooks were negative.

Wagner-Jauregg had recorded many successes, but there were also failures which were frustrating. The inoculated patient might show remission and seem cured, then months or even weeks later, a relapse would set in.

Then one day in 1917, an assistant brought in a case of a soldier from the Macedonian front, apparently the victim of malaria, and asked about the dosage of quinine to administer. Like a flash the idea occurred to Wagner-Jauregg that here was a chance to inoculate the paralytics directly with the blood of the infected instead of a serum. It was, of course, taking a great risk but the results warranted it. Nevertheless, mistakes were made. Sometimes the blood had not been examined microscopically and deadly parasites prevented the riddance of the fever, causing the patient to succumb. Bacteriologists, however, who were interested in their own problems, came to his aid and helped surmount some of the obstacles.

With a singleness of purpose characteristic of the man, the therapist expanded his method, experimenting in syphilis clinics, and in 1927, he was awarded the Nobel Prize. He might have received it years earlier, but the professor of psychiatry at the University of Stockholm could not bring himself to vote for a man who would add malaria to the already frightful condition of general paresis. In his eyes such a physician was simply a criminal.

Since the malaria treatment, other techniques have been devised to induce a high degree of humid heat, e.g., the cabinet (hypertherm) of Kettering or the use of a high-frequency electric current to raise the temperature of the patient.

Julius Wagner-Jauregg, the son of an Austrian official with a legal training, was born in 1857, in Wells, Austria. Even as a child, he was inclined to cut up cats to see what they were like inside. That he should choose medicine as a profession was hardly a surprise. Throughout his studies, he showed great promise as an experimentalist and received much encouragement from the famous professors at the University of Vienna, particularly Salomon Stricker. His promotion from assistant to Professor of Psychiatry was rapid.

Wagner-Jauregg looked Slavic rather than Teutonic. His grandmother was a Jauernick, and his father, upon his ennoblement, took on the name of Jauregg in her memory.

Sakel's Insulin Shock

It has often been remarked that discoveries are the results of propitious accidents; and yet it takes someone with an alert mind, in addition to fundamental training, to relate the chance happening to some scientific principle.

The Viennese physician, Manfred Sakel, was fortunate in the fact that one of his patients in Vienna had been given an overdose of insulin, which induced a stupor but later showed some remission of the symptoms. This circumstance marked the beginning of the shock therapies, just as Bertha Pappenheim's flow of memories under hypnosis set Freud on the road to formulating his system of psychoanalysis.

Sakel at first used insulin to treat alcoholics and drug addicts, then applied the technique to cases of schizophrenia. The procedure consists in administering intramuscularly increasing daily doses of insulin until the patient falls into a coma, in which he is kept for a variable period (from one-half hour to one hour usually). After a dextrose solution has been administered to restore the sugar loss, the patient shows signs of marked improvement in lucidity of speech and friendliness of attitude.

While Sakel reported a recovery rate of nearly 88 per cent of those receiving the treatment, much depends on the length of the period since the onset of the illness. There are also other factors, such as the age of the patient, the optimal decade being between twenty and thirty, auxiliary therapy along with the shock treatment, and the prepsychotic stability of the patient. In a number of cases, the patient does not respond, or if he does improve to the point of no longer being troubled by hallucinations or delusions, he may after a while sustain a relapse.

After Hitler's annexation of Austria in 1938, Sakel migrated to the United States, where, at the insistence of Commissioner F. Parsons, he introduced the treatment in New York hospitals. His work is described in *Pharmacological Shock Treatment of Mental Disease; Results of Shock Therapy,* and *Origin of Shock Therapy. The Philosophical Library* has brought out posthumously *Schizophrenia* and an uncompleted treatise on *Epilepsy,* with an introduction by Otto Poetzl, Sakel's former professor and now Director Emeritus of the Vienna Clinic, where the insulin shock therapy was first initiated.

Metrazol Shock

At about the same time that Sakel in Vienna was experimenting with insulin to produce convulsions in psychotics, Von Meduna (1896-   ) in Budapest, observing that schizophrenics who are also epileptic tend to show a remission of symptoms after their epileptic seizures, began to induce epileptoid seizures through drugs. Camphor had been known as an old stand-by in epileptic treatment, so Meduna used it in order to bring about the desired convulsions. When it did not prove satisfactory because of the difficulty in controlling the time element, he tried a camphor derivative called Metrazol.

This is injected intravenously. The *grand mal* convulsion which follows almost immediately is fraught with great distress and is not without possible danger, resulting in bone fracture due to the violent contraction of the muscles, so that curare is administered to counteract the too vigorous muscular activity. After the convulsion, the brief period of dread and confusion is followed by relaxed sleep. The shock serves to blot out some of the memories directly concerned with the psychotic condition.

A number of fatalities and grave consequences have been instrumental in lessening the wide use of Metrazol in favor of insulin therapy and electro-shock.

Metrazol therapy was tried out in a number of American hospitals, particularly before electro-shock appeared on the horizon. Several American journals and a number of books carried discussions of the treatment, led by Meduna's "General Discussion of the Cardiazol Therapy" in the *American Journal of Psychiatry*, Vol. 96, 1938.

L. Meduna migrated to the United States in 1939, when he took a post as associate professor at the Loyola University Medical School. His main works are *Convulsive Treatment of Schizophrenia*, 1938; *Histopathology of Epilepsy*, 1932; and *Carbon Dioxide Therapy*, 1950.

Electro-Shock

The electro-shock, which has become perhaps the most widely known therapy in the treatment of severe mental illness, was introduced by Ugo Cerletti (1877-   ) in 1938.

Cerletti, whose name is scarcely known even among psychiatrists, received his training under such men as Nissl and Kraepelin at Heidelberg. His research in both the normal and the pathological cell would have entitled him to some recognition, but he contributed also to the etiology of goitre and cretinism, and then began his studies on general paresis.

Cerletti's course had not been swift. He received impacts from various sources, including his teachers at the universities of Turin, Rome, Heidelberg and Paris. The electro-shock notion was the end-product of a long series of investigations, largely theoretical; and his decision to try out such a drastic therapeutic method as a shock precipitated through electricity was made late in life.

In some respects, the condition produced by the electro-shock, like an epileptic seizure with its brief period of unconsciousness, is much like that brought about by Metrazol. Here, too, there are similar dangers of fracture, which are minimized through the administration of curare. Electro-shock, however, despite a small number of fatalities, through cardiovascular failure and asphyxiation, is more expedient and effective than Metrazol therapy. Through it thousands of patients have found at least temporary relief, while some have shown remission of symptoms for long periods or even total recovery.

Various combinations of therapy have also been tried, such as insulin and electro-shock, narcosis and electro-shock—all still in the experimental stage. Standardized procedures are hardly to be expected because of the many variables in regard to the patient's constitution, severity of the case, and various other causes.

Cerletti, who worked in conjunction with L. Bini, later developed a serum from the brain of animals subjected to repeated electro-shock, containing what he called aeroagomines, which he considered vitalizing substances. An injection of this is calculated to do the same for the psychotic as the electro-shock without exposing him to the great discomfort and possibly disastrous aftermath of the earlier technique.

Moniz Cuts into the Brain

If the various shock treatments have had to contend with attendant peril to the patient, then brain surgery, developed by the Portuguese neuropsychiatrist, Egas Moniz, must be considered as the *ne plus ultra* of daring methods to relieve an unbearable condition.

Like most treatments, even this does not appear to be something *toto coelo* novel. Trepanning or perforating the skull would seem to have been practiced in the neolithic age.

To those of earlier generations, surgery meant the removal of pathological tissue, perhaps an infected area, or else the grafting of tissue or mending of impaired organs. But to cut away part of the very brain itself would have been thought madness until Egas Moniz electrified the world with his extraordinary treatment of patients suffering from hopeless depression.

There are two types of psychosurgery: (a) lobotomy, which means the severing of prefrontal lobe and thalamus, which governs the emotional system; and (b) lobectomy, which means the cutting away of parts of the prefrontal lobe, and not merely severing the nerve fibers as in lobotomy. Freeman and Watts, who introduced psychosurgery into the United States and elaborated on Moniz's original technique, performed the operation by driving a long instrument transorbitally into the white matter just above the eyeball.

Much has been written on these operations both pro and con. It is only in the most desperate cases, where the patient is in the very depths of depression and is entirely divorced from reality, that such procedures seem indicated. There have been some favorable results, of course, but aside from a certain percentage of mortality (variously reported as between 1 and 5 per cent), some of the higher-thought functions are irretrievably impaired. The chief gain is the relief of anxiety and the achievement of a certain composure by the patient, but often controls, both physical and mental, are lacking, judgment is unreliable, memory fades and the self or ego becomes more or less labile, in contrast with the previous affective tension.

There are definite personality changes. For one thing, the patient becomes more congenial, optimistic and energetic. If the intense suffering can be reduced through brain surgery without too great a loss in other directions and at no great risk, it seems worthwhile. If it is just a matter of revision of symptomatic outward behavior, then we must be chary of recommending it.

Egas Moniz (1874-1958), after gaining his medical degree, taught at Coimbra, Portugal, until 1911, and then became Director of the Institute of Neurology at Lisbon and Professor of Neuropsychiatry at the University there. His chief work was on cerebral angiography. It was in Lisbon that he developed the technique known as lobotomy or leucotomy, which proved more effective with melancholics than with schizophrenics. In 1949, he shared the Nobel Prize with Walter Hess.

III
EDUCATIONAL PSYCHOLOGY

E. L. THORNDIKE (1874-1949)—
The Pillar of Teachers College

If one were to name the leading educational psychologist in the United States over a period of decades, one would inevitably think of Edward Lee Thorndike, born in Williamsburg, Massachusetts in 1874. Educated at Wesleyan University and Harvard, where he came under the tutelage of William James, he received his Ph.D. at Columbia in 1898.

While still a young man, he published *The Human Nature Club,* a sort of popular textbook, already showing an individual slant. His early interest was animal psychology, and he devised controlled experimental methods which older animal psychologists like Romanes and Lloyd Morgan had not thought of. His box with levers arranged for cat experiments was one of his pioneer pieces of work.

In 1899, he was appointed instructor in genetic psychology at Teachers College, Columbia, serving as professor from 1906 and Director of the Psychology Division of the Educational Research Institute from 1922 to 1940. Easily the "big man" at Teachers College, he influenced thousands of students. His *Educational Psychology* (1903), expanded into three volumes, became a standard work in the United States. In 1904, he published *Mental and Social Measurements,* and in 1911 appeared *Animal Intelligence.*

He wrote on the psychology of mathematics and for a long period he was the oracle in educational statistical work, representing the multimodal view of intelligence and other personality components as against the unitary and bimodal theories (Spearman). Many were the controversies which his numerous articles aroused. He was also interested in tests for both school children and superior adults.

In later years Thorndike espoused studies along the lines of lexicography in connection with schools. Word frequency was the basis of his dictionary for children (1935) and one for young adults (1941).

Thorndike is known in psychology for his "theory of effect," according to which the satisfaction gained by an act tends to stamp it in, so that it will recur. The Associationist trend was strong in Thorndike.

A man of good address, he was courteous and correct in his transactions, popular with his students and one of the most productive American psychologists, having founded at Teachers College an important monograph series which incorporated the work of doctoral dissertations.

IV
TESTS AND MEASUREMENTS

LEWIS M. TERMAN (1877-1956)—
Ace of Test Specialists

Next to Binet, the name of Lewis Terman is most frequently associated with the psychological test movement. In fact, Terman devoted more years to the development of the Binet tests and became more of a specialist than Binet himself.

After attending the Central Normal College at Danville, he went to Indiana University, and then Clark University, which at the time was in its heyday so far as psychology is concerned.

In 1904, Terman took for his thesis the subject of mental testing. It was in the qualitative rather than the quantitative aspects that he was interested. It was not until his first year as assistant professor at Stanford University, in 1911, that he began his experimental study of the Binet tests, which resulted in the publication of *The Measurement of Intelligence,* in 1916. This at once became the standard work on the subject. A revised edition under the title of *Measuring Intelligence* appeared in 1937, under the joint authorship of Terman and Maud Merrill.

Terman undertook large projects with many assistants. His *Genetic Studies in Genius,* in three volumes, was a milestone in tracing the early development of the famous. The biographies of three hundred illustrious men and women were studied with a view of giving them an intelligence quotient, on the basis of their early letters, utterances, products, etc.

The results are sometimes startling and dubious, but the method is novel and the findings on the whole fruitful. The first of the volumes appeared in 1926, the last in 1948.

In *Sex and Personality,* Terman, in co-operation with Catherine Cox Miles, studied the essence of masculinity and femininity (1936) and in 1938 he brought out his *Psychological Factors in Marital Happiness.*

Terman was a champion of gifted children, and advocated not only special classes but special schools for them, later following up their careers.

Terman's standardization of the Binet (Stanford-Binet) Test became the household instrument of all institutions. For individual testing there has never been a better one. It was during the First World War that the importance of testing proved itself, and Terman's service was so great that he was regarded as the arbiter of all tests pertaining to the measurement of intelligence.

V
COLLECTIVE PSYCHOLOGY

HAYIM STEINTHAL (1823-1899)
Co-founder of Collective Psychology

While there have been many before Steinthal who reflected on the subject, it was he, together with his brother-in-law, Moritz Lazarus, who may be said to have founded the branch known as *collective* or group psychology.

Steinthal studied at the University of Berlin from 1843 to 1850, when he was appointed *Privatdocent* in philosophy and psychology. He was later, after a sojourn in Paris, named *Honorarprofessor,* which in Germany meant that he received *no* honorarium.

In psychology, both he and Lazarus were regarded as disciples of Herbart, but Steinthal had views of his own as well. Although his main interest was the philosophy of language, on which he was an authority, having studied Chinese and other remote languages, he made contributions to mythology, comparative religion, ethics, and logic, and naturally to psychology. His literary output was vast, and because his writings not infrequently met with opposition, he found himself engaged in polemics altogether too often.

It was his and Lazarus' "group mind" concept, in particular, that was attacked in academic circles. The doctrine that there was a group mind distinct from the collection of individual minds rendered him open to the suspicion that he believed in some mystical entity. In reality, however, Steinthal did not posit any supersoul or extra-individual mind hovering above the collective individuals, but understood the collective psyche to be an integration of the individual minds functioning as a unit under given circumstances.

Steinthal's style was facile but trenchant in controversy, as is indicated for example in the preface of his *Grammatik, Logik, und Psychologie* (Berlin, 1855). An erudite scholar, he was at the same time a social reformer. In his *Allgemeine Ethik* (Berlin, 1885), in which he discussed socialism and pleaded for absolute academic freedom and for the recognition of atheism as a religion, he evidenced a stage of liberalism and broad-mindedness unusual for a German professor of his time. In his *Principles of Psychology,* William James occasionally cites Steinthal as an authority.

GUSTAVE LE BON (1841-1931)—Polyhistor

Perhaps because of the too facile pen which he wielded sedulously for some seventy years out of the ninety which he was fortunate enough to live, this polyhistor is undeservedly either forgotten or shelved. But his numerous works, some of which were translated into at least a dozen languages and enjoyed edition after edition, were widely discussed and exercised a good deal of influence on the intelligentsia of two past generations.

Le Bon considered himself a psychologist and certainly he may be included among the social psychologists, but perhaps he was primarily a publicist with his plethora of ideas and opinions.

He wrote on a variety of subjects: tobacco smoking (1880); the evolution of matter; Arab civilization (a large tome with many colored plates); the civilization of India (an equally imposing volume); the evolution of force; the psychology of education; the psychology of socialism; political psychology; the psychology of revolution; the psychology of World War I; intra-atomic energy; the psychology of the evolution of peoples. The work, however, which went through more than a score of editions in French alone and which brought his name before the educated readers in many parts of the world was *The Crowd* (1897). His conclusions do not appear too original, but his vivid language and illustrations exerted an appeal. The crowd to him is more or less a bundle of emotions and acquires ideas only through contagion.

He was a bitter foe of socialism at a time when it was looked to as an ideal. Religion he viewed as a mass medium, believing the true soul of a people is revealed in its arts and institutions. His hostility to German values was on a par with his opposition to socialism. He did not believe in the ultimate results of progress. Indeed, he was skeptical of the existence of such a process, deeming it rather a convenient illusion.

ÉMILE DURKHEIM (1858-1917)
Founder of Sociological Methodology

Born into a middle-class Franco-Jewish rabbinical family at Épinal, Émile Durkheim completed his education in Paris, and after several teaching appointments and promotions, he was called to the Sorbonne, where, through his lectures and writings, he soon became known as the leading sociologist in France and, later, in Europe.

Not only was it to his credit that sociology became a full-fledged department of instruction in French colleges instead of a nook in philosophy, but his founding of the annual *L'Année Sociologique,* in 1898, opened up a new medium for those who were engaged especially in problems and issues that had been previously submerged.

The successor of Auguste Comte, he went much farther as an investigator, always fortifying his conclusions with facts, statistics, and ethnological data. Because of his ramified expansion in the social sciences and his growing prestige, it was inevitable that he should exercise some influence on psychology, as well as on the study of religion, anthropology, and even biology. His greatest contribution was to the field of labor distribution, particularly in its moral rather than economic aspect.

Not unlike the Jewish founders of collective psychology in Germany, Hayim Steinthal (*q.v.*) and Moritz Lazarus, he subscribed to a group mind which was not merely the summation but a transformation of the constituent individual minds. Through this collective phenomenon he sought to explain religious belief, various educational trends, and the authority of value judgments, which to him were of paramount importance. In all these works, the feeling of solidarity and the sentiment of social responsibility play a dominant part.

His solid works on the division of social labor, on sociological methodology, the latter of which has become a classic, on suicide, and on the elementary forms of religious life, have been translated into several languages, and he has left a host of ardent followers, mainly in France. His humanitarian work on behalf of the unfortunates during the First World War is scarcely known even in sociological circles.

LUCIEN LÉVY-BRUHL (1857-1938)

Born in Paris of Jewish parents, Lévy-Bruhl distinguished himself in his studies, and in his early forties became a professor at the Sorbonne. After the death of Ribot, he edited the *Revue Philosophique,* and in 1917 he was elected to the Académie des Sciences Morales et Politiques.

Lévy-Bruhl wrote mainly on the history of philosophy. His monographs on Leibniz, Jacobi, and Comte have been widely read. It was the latter, however, who exercised the chief influence on him, so that he may be considered a member of the positivist school. It was his aim to deal with the philosophical sciences, such as ethics, just as he would the natural sciences, thus anticipating the position of modern anthropology in its descriptive approach and ethical relativism.

He was often spoken of as the successor of Émile Durkheim, but they diverged in their views, the latter being more the sociologist with standards deriving from traditional molds, while Lévy-Bruhl was committed to a more anthropological and relativistic scheme of things.

Lévy-Bruhl will best be remembered by his books on primitive mentality, which date from 1910. *La Mentalité Primitive* and *L'âme Primitive* are his best-known works. The writer recalls how Lévy-Bruhl once entertained a gathering at the house of a Harvard professor with anecdotes about primitives—*e.g.*, how one of them asked a white resident reading a newspaper whether he was treating some eye trouble by holding the paper before his eyes. Primitive thinking, Lévy-Bruhl taught, is prelogical, centered on the supernatural and mystic. Primitive man does not perceive in the same way as civilized *homo sapiens,* although his nervous system is the same, and his sense organs may even function better. His milieu and experiences, however, are different; hence his interpretation, as in the case cited above, is warped.

The Theory of Evolution Looms

Bonnet was a contemporary of great naturalists who have made history. G. LeClerc Buffon (1717-1789), best remembered by a hyperbole on style (*Le Style est l'homme*), did outstanding work as a systematizer (*Histoire Naturelle*). However, he can in no way be compared with Georges Cuvier (1769-1832), who is remembered for his equally exaggerated assertion that an organism can be reconstructed from a single fossil bone on the premise that adaptation to the environment in order to survive shows in the shaping of all the organs toward a single goal.

The greatest naturalist of his day, Cuvier possessed a commanding personality which was recognized by royalty, including Napoleon. An indefatigable worker, he turned out volume after volume of his researches on fossil bones and (with a collaborator) on the natural history of fishes, which was to be completed in forty volumes.

The Transmission of Acquired Characteristics

Equally celebrated and of greater influence was J. B. Lamarck (1744-1829), propounder of the theory that acquired characteristics are transmissible as a result of efforts to adapt to conditions in order to survive. Lamarck's fame became widespread because of the controversies he precipitated. The chief opponent of his theory was August Weismann (1834-1914), who, by a series of carefully conducted experiments, proved to the satisfaction of most biologists that such acquisition is not transmitted from parent to child.

On the other hand, because of his "natural selection" principle Charles Darwin can be regarded as an ally of Lamarck; and he is often called a Neo-Lamarckian, since he supposed the continuation of achievement in a given species to be due to the fact that those of the progeny which inherited desirable traits survived while the others died out in the struggle for existence (but these traits could very well be chance happenings, not necessarily transmitted via the germ plasm). Of recent investigators who have endorsed Lamarck as against Weismann, the names of Paul Kammerer, in biology, and William McDougall, in psychology, may be mentioned, but their experiments have met with adverse criticism. In the USSR, the biological orientation of Michurin and Lysenko favors Lamarckianism.

The first half of the nineteenth century was a preparation period for the epoch-making message that Charles Darwin and Alfred Russel Wallace, together with a group of British supporters, were to bring to the world. Partly due to the universal interest in the doctrine of evolution and the polemics which it aroused, interest in animal psychology increased. In the same year that the *Origin of Species* appeared (1859) was born Jacques Loeb, who was to take up a position (tropism) on animals nearer to Descartes' mechanical view than to that of subsequent anthropomorphizers.

VI
ANIMAL PSYCHOLOGY

Contrary to general belief even among psychologists, animal psychology is not a recent branch. In an applied sense, there must have been animal psychologists even in Sumeria, some six thousand years ago, since managing camels or asses involved acquiring some knowledge of their behavior.

When we turn to Aristotle, we find a body of observations on the mind of animals which is truly astonishing. To be sure, from our present vantage point we can discern many naïve statements based on anecdote and hearsay, but the wonder is that this colossal thinker was able to gather so many data that are sound, indeed, that he should have seen any value at all in such a study. Lucretius, Horace, Seneca and Galen left observations on animals, but in general, with the exception of Lucretius's poetic insights, they were scant.

For many centuries after the classic period, animals seemed to have eluded the notice of the learned, who were too busy with their speculations about God and the soul and the cosmos to watch the dumb creatures. The great gulf that existed then between man and animals in the conceptual framework made the latter too inferior for theoretical consideration. In the bleak Middle Ages, we may at most glean a few references, proverbs, casual remarks relative to animals; and, of course, the various fables and bestiaries, all the way from ancient Aesop to masters like Lafontaine and Krilov, and the many versions of Reynard the Fox.

Such sophisticated elaborations as Goethe's *Reineke Fuchs* would indicate that animals always had their place in human thought, but they received no systematic investigation until recently.

One of the reasons—perhaps the main one—for the sharp separation between human and infrahuman organisms was the great role played by the implicit belief in the soul in directing our interests and values. Descartes found it awkward, if not absurd, to ascribe a soul to a cat or a dog; and since the soul was regarded as the basis of all feeling, it was only natural to deny the animal not only intelligence and will but even the capacity to feel. Hence, Descartes decided that an animal was an automaton; and his prestige was so great that even such a critical person as Salomon Maimon, as he tells us in his remarkable autobiography, kicked animals without compunction (at least in his youth) on the strength of Descartes' conclusion.

On the other hand, the fabulists always sought to humanize animals, making them think and talk and endowing them with human motives. They were depicted as prototypes of the shrewd and deceitful, the stupid, the irresolute, the impulsive, the foolhardy, etc.

It was not until the seventeenth century that "brutes" began to appear worth studying. The French, usually the first to pick up neglected causes, were in the *avant-garde* of the new movement, but the more intensive and objective work was subsequently done in Germany.

Considering the age, it is remarkable that so many field studies on insects, fish, earthworms, locusts, crickets, etc., appeared as early as the sixteenth century. De la Chambre's *Traité de la Connaissance des Animaux* appeared in 1662, Boullier's *Essai philosophique sur l'âme des bêtes* came out in 1728. Reaumier's *Histoire des Insectes* was printed in 1741, and Condillac published his *Traité des Animaux* in

1755. Georg F. Meier's *Seele der Tiere* appeared in 1756. But it was Hermann Samuel Reimarus who may be considered the first to give us a textbook on animal instinct in his *Allgemeine Betrachtungen über die Triebe der Tiere, hauptsächlich über ihre Kunsttriebe,* etc. (He drew out the title so as to link the whole with the "cognition of the relationship between the world, its creator, and ourselves.") Four editions of this work were brought out in a comparatively short time, and a French translation followed.

REIMARUS (1694-1768)

Reimarus, a professor of Oriental languages in Hamburg, was by virtue of his disciplined mind and extraordinary erudition well qualified to deal with the subject of animal psychology. His was a textbook in the modern style in that he cited the literature in several languages, and also because of his systematic development of the subject.

Not only did Reimarus present a large corpus of facts, some undoubtedly without much foundation; but, without sponsoring a theory of continuity like the exponents of evolution a century later, he did some close reasoning along the lines of biological adaptation to show why certain animals developed special sensory acuity and other useful means for survival.

He is generally concerned with proving that the arts of many birds and animals are not to be associated with intelligence, that the building of nests and weaving by spiders follow certain definite courses but are mechanical as compared with the evolution of the human arts, which are reflective. "The survival of the fittest" is implied in this work, and it is even possible to infer that Reimarus had some idea of "natural selection."

In one passage, he emphasizes the difference between man and beast by stating: "Nevertheless the ape remains an ape and between it and the most stupid person there is a greater separation than between the latter and a Leibniz or a Newon." [43] He refers to the fact that although the ape is an imitator, it cannot learn to keep a fire going from observing the behavior of humans. Commenting on this deficiency Reimarus writes: "It is perhaps fortunate that the apes show so little reflection and inventiveness. Unthinking as they are, they might have long ago set the American forests [*sic*] and plantations on fire and destroyed them." [44]

Reimarus was one of the independent thinkers of his age. A critic of dogmatic religion, he seemed close to British deism; and his discovery of a planned design in the arrangements of animal life would have placed him in the category of the teleologists. But whether he was a freethinker or deist, he could not bring himself to publish his work *A Defense of the Rational Worshipers of God,* in which all revealed religion is questioned searchingly.

After his death, his daughter Eliza, brought the MS to the attention of Ephraim G. Lessing, the critic and dramatist, who had become superintendent of the ducal library of Brunswick in Wolfenbüttel. In this capacity he had a right to publish worthy Mss found among the library treasures. Lessing's Jewish friend, the philosopher Moses Mendelssohn, whom he had consulted, advised against the publication, considering the work too radical and derogatory of the Christian Church, but Lessing published it under the title of *Fragments of an Unknown* as the literary remains of an anonymous author. It was published in fragments, each successive step being progressively bolder, until the resurrection of Jesus was impugned and shown to be an impossibility. Reimarus advanced a new slant on the purpose of Jesus, of which he took a dim view, representing him as a revolutionary who was imperiling the status of the country. He did not ascribe divinity to him but merely aggressive plans to establish himself as Messiah.

As could be imagined, an avalanche of denunciation fell upon the head of the great man of letters—perhaps the greatest in Germany at the time—and he was relieved of his post as library director. To get even with his revilers, he wrote *Nathan the Wise*, which is an effective plea on behalf of religious sanity and tolerance. The play did not appeal, of course, to the bigots and fanatics, but literary circles hailed it as a masterpiece.

Born in Hamburg in 1694 (December 22) Reimarus was fortunate in being educated by Fabricius, an eminent scholar, whose daughter he later married. His father had been a professor at a junior college; and after his studies at the University of Jena and a year's teaching at Wittenberg University, he became rector at the Wismar Gymnasium. In 1727, he occupied the chair of Oriental languages at Hamburg and stayed there until his death in 1768, declining a call to Göttingen. Everything he wrote had the stamp of scholarship and deep thought. Kant mentioned him as the greatest exponent of natural theology. Most of his works enjoyed many editions.

Despite his heresies in regard to revelation, the divinity of Jesus, the possibility of miracles and other dogmas, Reimarus did believe in an afterlife on the premise that the goal of man cannot be attained in a single lifetime, and as the soul is seeking perfection, and is a simple indivisible entity, it is constantly aiming to achieve perfection through perpetual evolution. Another argument for immortality is one which Kant later made the basis of his *Critique of Practical Reason*, viz., the law of justice in rewarding virtue and punishing wickedness.

Reimarus was an authority in several different fields; in the classics and in comparative psychology. As for Biblical history, let us bear in mind that the subtitle of the book which established Albert Schweitzer's reputation as a theological historian is *The Quest of the Historical Jesus, from Reimarus to Wrede.*

G. F. MEIER (1718-1777)

Another important pioneer in the history of animal psychology of whom little is now heard is Georg Friedrich Meier, a contemporary of Kant and, in his own day, quite influential both as a teacher and as a writer. Born in 1718 near Halle, he majored in theology and philosophy, and later taught philosophy. Although his chief work lay in the field of metaphysics, with a theological coloring, he was versatile and prolific in his output, writing also on literature and aesthetics and on animal psychology. One of his larger essays took up the question of German decadence in aesthetic matters. Psychology occupied a prominent position in his system of thought, and he considered the "soul" of animals in connection with the Cartesian denial that infrahuman organisms had any feeling whatever.

A disciple of Baumgarten, who was himself of the lineage of Wolff and Leibniz, Meier leaned toward the scholastic method of settling matters through argumentation. In 1744, he published his *Theoretical Doctrine of the Emotions,* and his theory (*Lehrgebäude*) in regard to the souls of animals came out in 1756.

Meier not only invested animals, and even insects, with intelligence but attributed reason to them, although on very flimsy grounds. His experiments were amateurish and his conclusions involved a begging of the question. He noted that when an ant came upon a dead fly and could not move it, except for half an inch or so, it disappeared; whereupon a fellow ant came along and tried to haul away the fly. In Meier's mind there was no doubt that the first ant communicated its difficulty to the other, and that this involved intelligent co-operation.

Ossa is piled upon Pelion in order to prove that the difference between man and animal is only one of degree; and that since the soul is the basis of man's mental life, the same must be said of the animal.

Actually, there is not much difference between Reimarus and Meier as regards their stand on the mental status of animals. The former is closer to us in method; the latter approaches the problem through reasoning. Both were in advance of their time in that they sought to remove the barrier between human and infrahuman existence and believed in a teleological dispensation. Meier was a theist, while Reimarus was a deist. That Meier wielded considerable influence in his day may be gathered from the fact that Kant thought well of him. In his precritical period, Kant could have passed for a follower of Baumgarten.

CHARLES BONNET (1720-1793)

One of the neglected men in the history of psychology is the Swiss naturalist, Charles Bonnet, whom we have earlier seen in the company of the French sensationalist, Condillac. Actually, they parted company on crucial issues. What they had in common was the scientific spirit, which held them aloof from anthropomorphism, as well as from Cartesian "mechanimalism" (if I may coin this portmanteau term). It is difficult to classify a complex character like Bonnet, who could be such a careful observer at the age of twenty-four that he discovered (to the astonishment of an established scientist, Réaumur) traces which served a certain insect as a guide to its nest after flights, while in later decades, he indulged in fantastic speculations about the soul worthy of a medieval scholastic (*La Palingénésie*).

It was because of his incongruous characteristics that Bonnet lost out in comparison with others who had less to their credit, but as an animal psychologist he was one of the early field workers and made several contributions not only to this field, but to botany and zoology. His paper on plant lice, published at the age of twenty, won him a corresponding membership to the Paris Académie des Sciences. When he was only twenty-four, he published a volume of papers under the title of *Insectologie,* which includes a scheme or scale of organisms that is on the borderline of the doctrine of transmutation of species.

As a botanist, he described the functions of leaves

and their use to the tree. His discovery of parthenogenesis and his experiments on polyps, worms, and spiders brought him to the fore in the zoological circle of the day. His grafting investigation (the head of one onto the trunk of another polyp), while primitive in the light of our modern techniques, stimulated research.

In physiology he anticipated the doctrine of specific nerve energies and sought the neural basis of memory, recognition, and attention. He also described a peculiar type of hallucination to which he was subject in advanced years.

That Bonnet should have turned to metaphysics and theology through teleological considerations, even defending the thesis that animals possess souls, is odd but not unique. We can think of Fechner, the founder of modern psychology, in the same connection. His readings of men like Leibniz must have affected him greatly, as Claparède suggests in his monograph; and a germinal mind which matures very early is sometimes apt to leap from one extreme to the other.

GEORGE JOHN ROMANES (1848-1894)
Comparative Psychologist

Canadian-born George J. Romanes was graduated from Cambridge University, in 1870, and after continuing his studies in France, Germany, and Italy, he returned to England where he carried out research on nerve irritability in Burdon Sanderson's laboratory at the University of London.

Although Romanes, who looked as if he might have had some gypsy blood, was known for his various stands on religion, changing from a somewhat atheistic to a rather deistic view, he was a pioneer animal psychologist. He applied the theory of evolution to comparative psychology, though he did not entirely exclude the anecdotal method from his scientific observations.

His *Animal Intelligence,* which appeared in 1881, was followed by *Scientific Evidences of Organic Evolution* in 1882, and *Mental Evolution in Animals* in 1883. In 1885, he brought out *Jellyfish, Starfish and Sea Urchins.* Then came *Mental Evolution in Man* in 1888. Subsequent books dealt with Darwinism and Weismannism.

To say, as Boring does in his *History of Experimental Psychology,* that "Romanes' book on animal intelligence is the first *comparative psychology* that was ever written" sounds a bit positive. He may have had a more scientific approach to the subject than his predecessors but Reimarus (*q.v.*) had already published a comparative psychology in Germany a century earlier. The first conscious approach to the study of comparative psychology in English, as Roback stated in 1920,[45] appears to be that of Romanes. Herbert Spencer, in the first article to appear in *Mind* (1876, vol. I), "The Comparative Psychology of Man," meant something different by this term, which only later came to connote the comparative method of investigating animal behavior. To Romanes, the term meant a comparison of the mental structures of organisms (including man), just as comparative anatomy dealt with their comparative bodily structures.

C. LLOYD MORGAN
The First Consistent Animal Experimenter

The first comparative psychologist in the modern sense was probably C. Lloyd Morgan. He advanced a step farther than Romanes, to whom, nevertheless, he acknowledges his indebtedness. His chief service was the introduction of the principle of parsimony—actually, the application to animal psychology of "Ockham's razor"—and there is no field in which this is more necessary, inasmuch as we tend to read into the behavior of animals our own purposes and motives.

In the preface to his *Comparative Psychology* published nearly seventy years ago, Morgan states, "I have laid much stress on the foremost importance of systematic and sustained observation as the only safe basis for conclusions concerning the intelligence of animals." His maxim throughout was that in dealing with animals we must take the simpler explanation first.

His systematic work is contained in *Animal Life and Intelligence* (1891) and *Habit and Instinct* (1896), both solid treatises in which the problem of nature and nurture is taken up at length, and in which he states his well-known position that acquired habits cannot be transmitted, as Lamarck and Darwin suggested. He does not believe that human intelligence as such has been growing through the ages but that advances in civilization are due solely to the storing and piling up of resources. Lloyd Morgan is inclined to discount much of what goes under the name of instinct and attributes behavior to habit based on environmental tradition or custom—a view akin to that of the anthropologists today.

In his *Animal Behavior* (1900), which is a rewritten revision of *Animal Life and Intelligence,* he deals largely with instinctive behavior and the social activities of bees and ants. Perhaps the most stimulating chapter is the one discussing animal "aesthetic" and "ethics." (The quotation marks are his, showing that he questions these designations.) Thus, he may be regarded as the first critical investigator in this branch of psychology.

When Romanes' sister thought her dog showed signs of shame by hiding his face after biting her, and then after more careful observation came to the conclusion that the animal's reaction was simply fatigue and listlessness after a bout of passion, Lloyd Morgan was pleased at the change of outlook. Similarly he attributes the apparent show of deceit on the part of a dog hobbling across the room, although it is not in the least injured, to the fact that "chance experience had led to a situation through which a hobbling gait had acquired the meaning of more petting and attention than usual."[46] Is this not an early formulation of Thorndike's law of effect?

Likewise he does not interpret the cat's play with the mouse before destroying it as an act of cruelty, a "torturing for torture's sake," but rather, as Groos theorizes, "The cat or kitten plays with the mouse not from innate cruelty but for the sake of getting some little practice in the most important business of cat life. Only man who has the capacity for nobler things can be cruel for cruelty's sake."

Philosophically, Morgan claimed to have been a monist, what we would call a psychophysical parallelist. He thought mind and body were the same, but experienced in a different manner.

Of greater moment was his doctrine of emergent evolution, which elicited much discussion in the fields of philosophy, psychology, and biology. Morgan taught that higher stages emerged from lower ones whenever the various elements somehow combined to produce a new formation. Thus consciousness emerged not by design or plan but by chance.

Morgan's approach to psychology was through zoölogy and geology, which he taught first. It was only after serving as professor in these at the University College in Bristol, England, that he turned to comparative psychology. Small wonder, then, that he should have taken such an earthy view of the animal mind, while others were anthropomorphizing it.

Entomological Studies

The so-called social insects—ants, bees, wasps—have had better luck in receiving the attention of comparative psychologists than many of the larger animals. Bonnet investigated molluscs, ants and spiders as early as 1740, more than a century before John Lubbock (later Lord Avebury) made his experimental findings on ants and bees (1882). A few years later (1887) insect experiments of Auguste Forel added to our fund of knowledge in this neglected area; and the following year, A. Binet published his conclusions on the psychic life of Microorganisms. Perhaps the man most associated with this type of work is J. H. Fabre (1823-1915), whose long life enabled him to turn out a mass of detailed observations.

The Jesuit Erich Wasmann's experiments with ants and other organisms were not always looked on favorably because of his uncritical interpretations of the behavior he observed. A. Bethe, in his German study (1898-1900) (*Must We Ascribe to Ants and Bees Psychic Qualities?*), goes to the other extreme. Ludwig Büchner's experiments with termites, bees, and beetles are among the best in the field. The specialist on ants was W. Morton Wheeler. In several impressive volumes he described the social life of the ant in such remarkable detail that one sometimes wonders whether interpretation did not advance far beyond description.

ROBERT M. YERKES (1876-1956)

If one were to single out the man who has done more than anyone else in the United States for comparative psychology, especially in the study of primates (chimpanzees, ourang-outangs, monkeys), that man would be Robert Yerkes.

Originally inclined toward medicine, he was guided into zoology, taking courses at Harvard under such distinguished men as Parker, Davenport and Castle, but afterward turned to philosophy and psychology under such great teachers as Palmer, James, Royce and Münsterberg. In 1907, appeared his book *The Dancing Mouse,* and he soon became an instructor at Harvard. His field was animal psychology, but the name he chose was *comparative psychology,* for he was primarily interested in methods of investigation.

As a teacher, he was not inspiring, but an occasional remark would startle his classes. Thus the present writer remembers his saying one day that a monkey, who, without training beyond observation, would use a hammer to drive a nail into a board might be called a genius, for the concept is only relative.

His *Introduction to Psychology* (1911) stressed the comparative angle, which he thought had been lost sight of.

He developed with associates a point scale of measuring intelligence which he thought might supersede the Binet scale. This was used to some extent in the examination of recruits during the First World

War, but the Stanford-Binet scale which Terman had developed had greater success.

Yerkes was President of the American Psychological Association and represented psychology in the National Research Council, and was also chief of the psychological division in the Surgeon-General's office.

In connection with this work, he brought out a nine-hundred-page quarto volume showing what psychology had contributed to the war service through the testing of 1,700,000 men and officers, the first time such an operation had been conducted on such a scale.

Yerkes stepped out of Harvard when he saw little prospect of promotion to a full professorship. He accepted the headship in psychology at the University of Minnesota, but later, when President Angell of Yale founded the Institute of Human Relations, Yerkes accepted the post of research professor, and worked for the establishment of a primate colony. After much effort and some frustration, he succeeded in realizing his project; and in Florida, he opened the Yale Laboratories of Primate Biology. The independently operated "Primate Eden in Florida" has since been named for its founder.

His reports, monographs and articles are not well known, but his greatest, *A Study of Anthropoid Life,* upon which his wife collaborated, remains a standard work.

Yerkes was an excellent organizer and was looked up to in council halls, where he exerted considerable influence. A promoter of psychology at a time when it was still regarded as an adjunct of philosophy, he nevertheless takes rank as an able investigator. Although he worked with John B. Watson in developing methods of visual discrimination in animals, he could never accept the doctrine of behaviorism.

North America began to take the hegemony in animal psychology long before her importance in other fields of psychology became established. It was in the first decade of this century that E. L. Thorndike introduced new techniques in animal experimentation which ruled out subjective approaches. Thorndike worked with cats, but it was not long before the rat became the most frequently seen animal in psychological laboratories—the standby that continues to yield the most results. Monkeys, from anthropoid apes to the macacus rhesus, have been the subject of fascinating studies by Yerkes, Hamilton and Kellog, to name a few.

During the last decade E. C. Tolman at the University of California applied the results of hundreds of rat experiments to human behavior, and at Harvard University B. F. Skinner has been working patiently and extensively with pigeons, as well as with other organisms. O. M. Mowrer has conducted some interesting experiments with Australian birds, teaching them to talk and sing.

EPILOGUE

Lovers of animals, whether cats, dogs, horses or apes, are tempted to impute to them various qualities which are contestable. The famous case of the Elberfeld horses, who were supposed to be able to count, spell, and even guess correctly, is well known.

In his autobiography, Martin Freud tells of his sister Anna's dog Wolf getting lost after a fright and later jumping into a cab and raising his "nose sufficiently high to permit the taximan to read his name and address on the medallion hanging from his collar: 'Professor Freud, Berggasse 19.'"[47]

On the same page we read of a yet more canny sense attributed to a dog. Sigmund Freud's chow Jofi was such a good judge of character that "the whole family including Paula, our faithful maid, showed considerable respect for her canine sensibility. When the dog condescended to be stroked, the visitor enjoyed the best possible introduction. If Jofi, for instance, sniffed somewhat haughtily around the legs of a caller and then stalked off with a touch of ostentation, there was at once a strong suspicion that there was something wrong with that caller's character. Contemplating Jofi's selective qualities at this distance of years, I feel bound to admit that her judgment was most reliable."

In this connection, it is interesting to note that Ernest Jones, in his monumental biography of Freud, felt that the master was a poor judge of human character, and when I was impelled to query this, Jones wrote me that there was no question about the fact, and that Freud was aware of this deficiency in himself. That a chow would be a better judge of human character than the founder of psychoanalysis is a proposition hard to swallow.

The incommunicability of the more intelligent animals is something that lends itself to romantic interpretations. In recent weeks, a news item has appeared about a bloodhound which led the police to an escaped prisoner, who was promptly returned to a cell, where the dog was seen to lick him affectionately. It would be natural to read into the dog's act a feeling of remorse or a desire to compensate, but most likely the dog did not reflect on the difference between a criminal and an honest citizen and may have simply looked upon him as a poor soul lost in the bushes who needed sympathy.

Actually, we can never know what the dog felt, or to what extent the feeling or sentiment took any clear shape, or whether it was just a momentary attraction, especially if the dog were female, and the prisoner of the agile, motor type.

FOOTNOTES

1. Transl. by E. A. Quain.

2. This does not sound right. "Into which" would make better sense. A.A.R.

3. St. Augustine: *Confessions,* transl. by N. J. Bourke, Fathers of the Church, Inc., pp. 351-352.

4. Hans Gruhle, a distinguished psychiatrist, was a sympathizer rather than a votary—perhaps more a patron, figuring on the editorial board of the journal.

5. C. Spearman: *History of Psychology in Autobiography* (ed. by Murchison), Vol. I.

6. A. A. Roback, *A History of American Psychology* (Library Publisher), 1952, p. 141.

7. E. G. Boring, in *History of Psychology in Autobiography* (ed. by C. Murchison), Vol. 4, pp. 32-33.

8. *History of Psychology in Autobiography* (ed. by C. Murchison), Vol. 2, p. 376.

9. D. B. Phemister, "The Transmission and Recovery of Greek and Roman Medical Writings," in *The Albert Schweitzer Jubilee Book* (ed. by A. A. Roback), p. 347.

10. E. W. Taylor, "Medical Aspects of Witchcraft," in *Problems of Personality* (ed. by A. A. Roback), p. 181.

11. H. W. White, *Demonism Verified and Analyzed,* p. 15.

12. J. Sprenger and H. Kraemer, *Malleus Maleficarum* (trans. by M. Summers), p. 109.

13. *Ibid,* p. 112-113.

14. *Ibid.*, p. 114.

15. *Ibid.*
16. *Ibid.*, p. 117.
17. *Ibid.*, p. 121.
18. *Ibid.*, p. 226, col. 2.
19. A. Stoddart, *The Life of Paracelsus*, London, 1911.
20. C. G. Jung, *Paracelsica*, Zürich, 1942.
21. R. M. Lawrence, *Primitive Psychotherapy and Quackery* (Houghton Mifflin, 1910), p. 246.
22. Jean Wier, *Histoires et Disputes des Illusions et Impostures*, Vol. I, p. 482. This is a reprint of the old French translation of *De Praestigiis*. Apparently there is no modern French translation.
23. G. Zilboorg, *History of Medical Psychology* (Norton), p. 228.
24. A. Lemoine, *Le Vitalisme et l'Animisme de Stahl.*
25. G. Zilboorg, *History of Medical Psychology* (Norton), p. 294.
26. R. Burton, *The Anatomy of Melancholy*, Part I, Sect. 2, Memb. 2, Subs. 4.
27. E. Haskell, *Trial of Ebenezer Haskell in Lunacy and His Acquittal*, pp. 98-100. Haskell's account of his own experiences reads like fiction.
28. Ph. Pinel: *Traité Médico-Philosophique sur l'Aliénation Mentale*, 2d ed., 1809.
29. *J. Guislain, Leçons orales sur les Phrénopathies*, 2d ed. (ed. by B. C. Ingels), 1890, Vol. I, p. 108.
30. *Loc. cit.*, Vol. 2, p. 360.
31. His *Traité sur l'Aliénation Mentale*, 1826, was held in high regard by continental specialists.
32. Since "credulity" has already become the established term for normal gullibility, it would seem that "credivity" should be the term applied to the abnormal condition of belief found in the psychotic. Belief is the word for the ordinary condition.
33. W. B. Carpenter, *Principles of Human Physi-*

ology, 1852. Part of this was amplified and published separately as *Principles of Mental Physiology.*

34. H. Maudsley, *The Physiology and Pathology of the Mind,* 1867.

35. P. J. Möbius, *Ueber die Anlage zur Mathematik,* 1907.

36. E. Kraepelin, *Lehrbuch der Psychiatrie,* 8th ed., 1913, Vol. III, p. 669.

37. E. Kraepelin, *Psychiatrie,* 8th ed., 1913, Vol. I, p. 704.

38. G. C. Ferrari, *History of Psychology in Autobiography,* Vol. II, p. 71.

39. S. De Sanctis, *History of Psychology in Autobiography,* Vol. III, p. 96.

40. M. Nordau, Degeneration, 8th English ed., 1896, Book III, Chapt. 1, p. 254.

41. W. Muncie, *Psychobiology and Psychiatry* (Mosby), p. 29.

42. For more details, see A. A. Roback: *Psychology of Character,* 3rd ed., 1952 (chapter on "Compensation").

43. Thomas Huxley, the enthusiast of the doctrine of continuity in evolution, thought that the gap was between man and man.

44. H. S. Reimarus: *Ibid.* 3rd ed. (1773) p. 254, ch. 9.

45. Roback: "The Scope and Genesis of Comparative Psychology" *J. Philos. Psych. & Scient. Method,* 1920, vol. 19.

46. C. Lloyd Morgan: *Animal Behavior,* London, 1900, p. 280.

47. Martin Freud: *Glory Reflected* (Angus and Robertson) London, Sydney, pp. 191-192.

INDEXES

REGISTER OF PERSONAL NAMES (NAMES IN QUOTES ARE PSEUDONYMS OR OF MYTHICAL CHARACTERS)

C

D

T

U

V

W

Y

Z

INDEX OF TOPICS